Intermittent Fasting for Women over 50

2 Books in 1

The Ultimate Guide to Accelerate Weight Loss, Promote Longevity, and Increase Energy with a New Lifestyle, Metabolic Autophagy and Tasty Recipes.

Table of Contents

Intermittent Fasting for Women Over 50

The simple guide to understanding your nutritional needs as a mature woman through the process of metabolic autophagy, support hormones and anti-aging boosters

Introduction

What Is Intermittent Fasting?

Intermittent fasting is not a diet, but a type of diet and lifestyle. The basic principles of intermittent nutrition, differences, and advantages over diets for weight loss, benefits for the body.

Intermittent fasting is a nutritional scheme with food breaks lasting 16-24 hours. The second name is a sinusoidal diet, but to call such a diet a diet in the broad sense of the word will be wrong. Food breaks are not a diet, but a type of food that has become a way of life for many people. Intermittent nutrition is compared to eating because it is often used for weight loss, but this system has several advantages over traditional diets.

Any diet for weight loss will be designed for a certain period, if you adhere to a diet longer than the specified time, it will lose effectiveness, as the body will have time to get used to it and slow down the metabolism. Exceeding strict diets can be hazardous to health. After completing the diet, the weight inevitably returns; this will happen even if the calorie content of the diet after the diet does not increase. Not everyone can afford to follow a diet since many do not withstand strict food restrictions for a long time. Mono-diets are not only challenging to tolerate but also represent a health hazard; for example, popular protein diets negatively affect the kidneys.

Intermittent fasting is more beneficial than traditional diets for weight loss. This system can be adhered to for many years, while addiction and the metabolic slowdown will not occur. Nutrition will remain complete, the body will not suffer from a lack of nutrients, as is the case with mono-diets.

The intermittent power system involves several schemes to choose from, so people have the opportunity to select the type of power that suits them.

Sticking to intermittent fasting is not as difficult as it might seem at first glance. With the right choice, a suitable scheme will not require tremendous willpower and continuously struggle with hunger. Intermittent or every other day nutrition provides all the benefits that fasting brings, first of all, it is healing and rejuvenation. In all nutritional schemes, the fasting period does not last longer than a day. This period is enough for the body to switch to internal nutrition, from a medical point of view, this is not starvation, as it occurs just 24 hours after the last meal.

Efficiency from intermittent fasting depends on the lifestyle that a person leads. In the periods between food breaks, the diet will not be limited by anything. This food system does not imply the separation of products into harmful and useful, permitted, and forbidden. Compliance with intermittent fasting does not require preliminary preparation; restrictions after refusing such nutrition are also not provided.

Intermittent Power Benefits

- **The ability to choose a power system at convenient intervals for yourself, from 16 to 24 hours.**

- **The frequency of pauses can also be different - every other day, once a week or once a month, it depends on the goals of the person.**

- **During periods of abstinence from food, you can drink water in unlimited quantities.**

- **You can adhere to such a regime for a very long time; it does not harm health.**

- **The availability of adaptation, at the very beginning, food breaks can be carried out once a month, then - with a denser frequency.**

- **No restrictions on food, no preferred products. Absolutely everyone can adhere to an intermittent diet - raw foodists, people on separate meals, vegetarians, and vegans.**

Is Intermittent Fasting Good for Older Adults

If you have not paid attention, intermittent fasting is still hot. Powered by recent research, it is developed with the help of many popular health and fitness magazines, websites, and blogs. But is intermittent fasting a good strategy for 50+ adults? We explore this question here.

What Is Intermittent Fasting?

Intermittent fasting term (IF) can be applied to any number of different dietary protocols. Unlike —true‖ fasting, where no calories are consumed for some time, intermittent fasting often allows for some calories on –fasting‖ days, and those days are the usual –feed‖ days.

Are associated with Alternate days include daily ADF (0 to 25%) of daily caloric intake, usually between meals. 5: 2 If the diet is the same, except that 25% of calories are consumed only on two unexpected –fast‖ days each week, the other five are usually fed.

Finally, there is a time-limited feeding (TRF), which is not fasting fast, but where ordinary foods are kept relatively short for short periods (for example, 10 am to 6 pm). In between), on an ongoing basis.

What's All the Fuss About?

If a quick scan of the latest literature on IF reveals that this relatively simple dietary strategy can prevent or cure anything. According to sampling book titles on Amazon, intermittent fasting can help you: Lose weight, build muscle, increase your metabolism, reduce fat, improve your memory, your body Fix, and be more productive. Although many of these claims may seem familiar to anyone who has ever tried the Poor Diet, the research behind these bold book titles holds little promise.

Still, experts caution that there are potential risks. Fasting can be dangerous for people with diabetes or other conditions where maintaining a constant level of blood glucose is essential. Avoiding eating during exercise can lower blood sugar, which can cause dizziness, lightheadedness, and confusion. And for those who take medicines for heart disease and hypertension, fasting can lead to dangerous electrolyte imbalances.

What the Science Says

Scientists have been studying fasting and mealtime protocols for decades, but in recent years, as more sophisticated methods have been implemented, the field has exploded.

The current buzz is the result of many studies that have not only improved weight loss but also improved metabolic factors such as insulin resistance and lipid profiles, as well as preventing academic decline, fighting cancer, and slowing down the aging process.

Have shown favorable results. General Chat Lounge Interestingly, most of these studies have been performed on laboratory animals (such as mice and insects), and almost all human trials have been relatively short-lived, with small sample sizes.

The results of the somewhat more fantail annual human trials were considered disappointing for this field - if it helped people lose weight and improve their lipid profiles. Still, it did less than usual calorie weight loss protocols. It didn't work any better. Also, subjects in the IF group had the highest dropout rates (13 out of 34), and the most common reason for quitting was the difficulty of staying on the protocol.

This is in stark contrast to the initial studies that showed a much higher rate of adherence to the IF protocol when the trial time was reduced (for example, eight and 12 weeks). Although more research is needed to determine if and how IF and TRF can be beneficial, researchers and other experts agree that this is an essential source of the fight against obesity.

As one literature review successfully stated, —Ultimately, it is the degree of adherence and stability of the diet, rather than the type of dietary strategy that will predict the consequences of weight loss.‖ In other words, people are different, and some people find it easier to eat more time than fasting or with a time limit. Some studies suggest that people who follow the TRF protocol lost weight despite being instructed to eat —ad libitum‖ or not.

Firsthand Experiences

Registered nutritionist Sharon Lahr man, nutrition, health, and fitness owner in St. Louis Park, Minn., Recommends fasting for her clients, about 70 percent of whom are over 50 years old. She uses something similar to 5: 2. If the protocol, —Mainly with people who have already lost weight, and we are using it more for recovery.‖

Why not lose weight? -This can be effective,‖ he said. However, it is prolonged. –It's going to be a pound a week,‖ says Lehmann. Lehman also agreed with researchers that what works for one person may not work for another. —There isn't a high diet. People can lose weight and maintain weight on different eating patterns.

So, it makes sense to work with people where they are.‖ Klein smith tried to limit his diet from time to time to improve his diet and hoped to take advantage of some of the long-term benefits of IF. It seems natural to restrict from noon to eight o'clock in the afternoon.

—It changes how you talk about food —If you're hungry, you don't always have to run and get something to eat.‖ After practicing RF, she lost about seven or eight pounds. (Losing weight was not the primary motivation for trying her diet.)

How to Eat During Menopause

Hundreds of years ago, few survived to menopause. Thanks to the development of medicine, the improvement of living conditions, and the abundance of food, life expectancy has almost doubled. It is worth using this gift and maintaining a high quality of life.

Although the term –menopause‖ itself is well known, many do not know how to cope with emerging problems and do not always receive satisfactory answers to improve their quality of life.

The Hebrew term —transitional age‖ is inaccurate. Our whole life is a transitional age from one period to another, and changes occur throughout life. The most appropriate Latin term is —menopause.‖

Nowadays, the biological age of many women is significantly lower than the passport, and yet many of them menopause causes all kinds of unpleasant phenomena. Different women have different menopause, but there are standard features of its manifestations.

On average, menopause occurs in 50-52 years, but age varies among different women. Menstruation may stop immediately, or their extinction will last for several months with an increase in the interval between them. During this period, you can make a simple blood test for the follicle-stimulating hormone FSH, which will distinguish menopause from its previous changes. If the hormone level is high, we are talking about menopause. If low - menstruation will continue.

What Are the Symptoms of Menopause and How to Deal with Them?

There are some symptoms which briefly describe below.

- **Weight gain**
- **Anatomical changes**
- **Sleep disturbances**
- **The tides**
- **Dry vagina and soreness of intercourse**
- **Frequent urination due to hypersensitivity of the bladder**

Weight Gain

It can occur without changing eating habits, due to a decrease in metabolic rate. Therefore, it is recommended to create a new nutritional program. You can lose weight at this time, but it will be more difficult, and the main goal is to maintain current weight without getting fatter.

It is now known that at this age it is advisable to weigh a little more, and not less, it is essential not only for appearance but also for health. Too rapid weight loss can cause the breakdown of muscle (sarcopenia) and bone (osteopenia and osteoporosis) tissues, as well as sagging skin of the neck and face.

I repeatedly explain to my patients older than 50 that if you lose weight, then slowly and gradually, accompanying the process with heavy drinking (8-10 glasses a day of any liquid without sugar, instead of which you can use artificial substitutes or stevia). In some cases, in general, I do not recommend losing weight but switch to a healthy diet.

It is advisable to engage in physical education - this is useful to everyone. Slow weight loss maximizes the preservation of facial skin quality and slows down muscle breakdown, which is very important. You cannot go on strict diets; 20 years of age still will not return.

What to eat? For such cases, a bread diet is well suited. The nutrition program is selected individually based on a blood test, a medical history, and external signs of nutrient deficiency. This includes building a diet, nutritional coaching, if necessary, taking dietary supplements.

Anatomical Changes

If there were problems with the hips before, now the fat begins to be deposited on the stomach. This is not only an aesthetic problem, but abdominal obesity also increases the risk of diabetes, hypertension, cardiovascular diseases, etc. Prevention - proper nutrition (a bread diet has a beneficial effect on the waist circumference) and physical education.

Sleep Disturbances

They develop in many women during menopause, including difficulty falling asleep, waking up in the middle of the night, after which it is difficult to fall asleep, and an early rise. Some women have difficulty sleeping 3-4 hours at night. It is essential to understand that this problem requires urgent treatment.

Lack of sleep causes fatigue, decreased tone, and a tired appearance. Also, it contributes to weight gain, the development of diabetes, and other health disorders.

There are various treatments. Relaxation, biofeedback, and other alternative medicine can help someone. Still, often you need to take drugs starting with natural, based on extracts of valerian, lemon balm, passionflower, and other plants that are sold over the counter and help to cope with sleep problems during menopause. Sometimes you have to resort to prescription drugs.

It is believed that drugs for insomnia are addictive, and many women, because of this, refuse to take them. But most modern medicines are neither addictive nor overwhelmed nor headaches in the morning.

Worth mentioning is the ―hormone of darkness‖ melatonin, the dosage form of which is called ―Circadian.‖ It can very well help with sleep problems - on its own or in combination with other medicines.

It is recommended to sleep at night for 7-8 hours, which will help to be in good shape and maintain a youthful appearance and clarity of thought. Daytime sleep cannot wholly replace nighttime sleep.

The Tides

This is a common phenomenon during menopause that can be cured. Hot flashes reduce the quality of life for many years. Hormones can help, but they are even more feared than sleeping pills. Why?

This is partly because several years ago, a publication was published that supposedly hormone replacement therapy increases the risk of breast cancer and cardiovascular disease. Despite the fact that it was proved that the research methodology was incorrect, the fear remained both among doctors and among patients. It's a pity. Today it is clear that hormone therapy helps with most problems caused by menopause, literally on all points from this article, except, perhaps, weight changes, but hormones can sometimes help with weight problems.

There are women to whom such treatment is contraindicated, and they need other methods. You need to consult with a specialist in menopause and decide with him whether it is possible to be treated with hormones and whether it is worth it. Hormones are taken in the form of tablets, skin stickers, as well as gel or tablets introduced into the vagina.

In addition to hormones, some plants help to cope with the tides, for example, racemose. Worth trying Nowadays, antidepressants are also used to combat hot flashes, but most of them increase appetite and promote weight gain.

Dry Vagina and Soreness of Intercourse

This is a common problem that is difficult to cure. Hormone therapy can also help here. Also, there are non-hormonal drugs that improve the situation, for example, a gel that is injected into the vagina before intercourse.

This is a simple method, but, unfortunately, many women do not know that KY gel and its analogs used for lubrication increase moisture in the vagina during intercourse. Lubricant gels are sold in pharmacies without a prescription.

Another gel, Binominal, contains hyaluronic acid. It must be administered daily, and it is also sold over the counter. Alas, not everyone knows about him, but he significantly improves the quality of life without any side effects.

Dry vagina not only overshadows the marital life but also increases the risk of cystitis.

Frequent Urination Due to Hypersensitivity of the Bladder

Most often, this manifests itself at night, but not only. Learning to control and strengthen the pelvic muscles using biofeedback, special exercises, as well as electrotherapy, and medications can help to cope with the problem. A particular treatment method is suitable for every woman, but they are not always told about the availability of different ways, and they do not ever complain about the problem.

Anticholinergics are most commonly prescribed. They have measurable minor side effects - mainly dry mouth.

All of the above is general advice, and in each case, you should visit a doctor, maybe even more than once, following existing problems.

In conclusion, I'll say that it's not necessary to suffer during menopause, you need to check, ask, find out and look for the best specialists to treat each problem, but there are such specialists. You can turn menopause into a great time in life.

Does Intermittent Fasting Make You Look Younger?

Individuals who want to be healthy and look younger can see the effects of intermittent fasting. There is further evidence that such intermittent fasting has weight gain and anti-aging benefits. Eating just a light meal can help you to avoid diseases and control these wrinkles. According to new research, people who ate a low-calorie diet for five days a month have lower cholesterol levels, blood pressure, and body fat.

On average, dieters shed five pounds on a diet three months later, and they see better control of blood sugar, reducing the risk of diabetes. Also, they have found little evidence of inflammation, a significant predictor of cancer, heart disease, and obesity. Intermittent fasting is called a fast copying diet based on a specific product line that provides up to 750-1,100 calories a day with small-scale nutrition such as food bars, soup packets, and tea. Victor Longo and colleagues at USC's Longevity Institute published this research in the Science Translation Medicine journal.

He explains that dietary cycles have reduced body weight, blood pressure, blood sugar, and body fat and have not had severe adverse effects. Another study, focusing on the impact of the dietary overdose, says that they have observed that a monkey showed a significantly longer lifespan after dieting. The age of the primate was started at the age of 16 at a 30% calorie restriction diet, which is equivalent to the late middle age for this type of animal.

Now, at 43 years old, monkeys have broken the longevity record for this species, which equates to about 130 in human years, according to a Scientific American report. Studies have repeatedly shown that intermittent fasting, or eating a small amount of food, can prolong life. However, the articles in these studies have been nematodes or primate diseases.

Another research, published this week in Science Translational Medicine, suggests that animal results can translate well into humans, with fasting three months at regular intervals only five days a month. The results can be useful in reducing the risk factors for aging.

Scientific or Evidence-Based That Intermittent Fasting Makes You Look Younger?

One of the most well-known ideas of aging includes the liberal ideology that emerged in the 1950s. The independent theory of aging describes that the biological age because cells accumulate independent underlying damage over time. Free radicals are any atom or molecule that contains only one pair of electrons in the outer shell.

The Free Radical Theory states, —If there are too many free radicals in our body, then free radicals will damage the cell wall, destroying the cell wall.‖ Fasting is powerful in protecting the cell wall. Cell walls can be retained as free radicals disappear or decrease by fasting.

So intermittent aging will reduce aging. Scientists have examined how fasting affects cellular and mitochondrial function and longevity. They have found that the cells of our body are fasting in the same way that they exercise. When stressed, cells - exercise or fast - react to changes at the cellular level that help to age us.

What Is The Ideal Time For Intermittent Fasting?

We'll take two widely accepted healthy eating —rules‖ and twist them in our head:

Rule 1: You Have To Eat First Thing In The Morning:

Make sure you start with a healthy breakfast. So, you can have it. First, firing metabolism in the morning! —Eat breakfast like a king, have lunch like a prince, and eat like a bandit.‖ There are even studies that show people who eat on the first day lose more weight than those who ate or skipped meals later in the day.

Rule 2: Eat Lots of Small Meals to Lose Weight:

Make sure you eat six small meals throughout the day so that your metabolism stays maximal throughout the day. In other words, —Eat breakfast and lots of small meals to lose weight and gain maximum health.‖ But if there are science and research that demonstrates skipping BREAK (excellent! Humiliating messenger) then it helps maximize human performance, improve mental and physical health, maintain more muscle, and lose fat in the body Can you?

That's Where an Intermittent Fasting Plan Comes In.

Fasting is not a diet but a diet. Put: it is making a conscious decision to skip certain foods according to the purpose. Fasting and then eating deliberately, intermittent fasting usually means that you feed your calories during a particular window of the day and do not eat for a large window of time.

Intermittent Fasting 16/8-time plan?

Fasting for 16 hours and then eating only in a specific 8-hour window. For example, eating alone at 8 pm, essentially skipping breakfast. Some people eat alone in a 6-hour window or even a 4-hour window. It is the –feast‖ and –fast‖ of your days and is the most common form of intermittent fasting. It's also my favorite way (lasting four years).

You Can Adjust This Time to Work for Your Life:

- If you start eating at 7 am, skip meals and start fasting at 3 pm.
- If you start eating at 11 am, skip the meal and start fasting at 7 pm.
- If you start eating at 2 pm, skip meals and start fasting at 10 pm.
- If you start eating at 6 pm, stop eating and start fasting at 2 am.

Intermittent Fasting Thing 24 Hour

Skip two meals a day, where you take 24 hours off from your feed. For example, eat on a regular schedule (ending dinner at 8 pm) and then by 8 am the next day you are not eating again. With this plan, you eat your usual three meals each day, and then occasionally choose breakfast and a day to skip lunch the next day. If you can only do 18 hours faster, or 20 hours faster, or 22 hours faster - that's fine! Adjust with different time frames and see how your body reacts. Two examples: skipping breakfast and lunch one day a week, and then another where you skip lunch and dinner one day, two days a week.

These are two of the most intermittent fasting plans, and we'll focus on those two, though there are several variations you can edit yourself:

- Some people eat in a 4-hour window. Yes, others do 6 or 8.
- Some people fast for 20 hours or fast for 24 hours.
- Another strategy is to have only one meal a day (OMAD).

You will need to experiment, adjust to your lifestyle and goals to work, and see how your body reacts.

Should I Eat Small Meals A Day?

There are a few main reasons why diet books recommend small meals:

1) When you eat food, your body needs to burn extra calories to process this diet. So, the theory is that if you eat with small meals all day, your body is always burning extra calories, and your metabolism is firing at maximum capacity. Well, that's not true. Whether you eat 2000 calories a day or 2000 calories in a small window, your body will burn the same number of calories the food is processed. So, the whole —always keep your metabolism at maximum efficiency‖ sounds good in principle, but reality tells a different story.

2) When you eat small meals, you are less likely to overeat during regular meals. I can see some truth here, especially for those who struggle with pest control or don't know how much to eat. However, once you educate yourself and control your diet, some will find that eating six times a day is very prohibitive and requires a lot of hard work.

I know I do. Also, since you are eating six small meals, I would argue that you probably never feel —full,‖ and you may want to consume extra calories during each breakfast. Although based on logical principles, —eating six meals a day‖ doesn't work because you think it is, and generally works only for people who Struggle with part control.

If we think about humans, if we have to eat every three hours, we as a species would have to face severe problems. Do you think Joe Kilian pulled out pocket pendants six times a day to eat equal amounts of food?

Chapter 1:
How Does Intermittent Fasting Work?

Myths of Intermittent Fasting

Myth 1: "You Will Always Feel Hungry"

A fictional tale of the fasting regimen. If there ever was a false lie about fasting, then this is the biggest.

Intermittent fasting is not a starvation diet, but a healthy lifestyle and an informed choice. You decide when it can begin and end. The point of the post is that you have full control over this.

He who is starving does not fast. They cannot control when it is time for the next meal or when starvation ends. Starving one does not consciously choose this.

Intermittent Fasting Is Not The Same As Fasting.

The average person is not going to starve, much less go into starvation mode if he does not have enough food. Think about it: if you eat 21 times a week, for 52 weeks a year. That is, you have 1092 meals a year.

Do You Think This Is the Right Approach to Your Health?

If you think that if you will starve for 24 hours - even once a week throughout the year, does your body starve at 18 meals (instead of 21)?

For math enthusiasts, this equals 928 meals versus 1092, annually. To further debunk this myth. Then think about the fact that in a state of fasting, your metabolism rises. That is, when you fast, you burn even more calories. MORE, no less.

With more extended starvation, adrenaline rises, which leads to an increase in metabolism.

The idea is that when you stop eating. Your metabolism falls and goes into this mythical state of hunger, just not right. This is the exact opposite! According to the results of studies with 4-day fasting, metabolism increases by 12%. Interestingly, when we try to limit calories in an attempt to lose weight, we see the opposite.

When someone begins to limit calories, it slows down. Therefore, because of this, the ability to lose weight is reduced.

Myth 2: Fasting Causes Muscle Exhaustion.

Let me put it very clearly here to make it clear. 2 types of energy stores in our body: sugar or fat. Thus, the body can use only two forms of energy that it stores. Which, as you probably guessed, is sugar or fat.

The proteins that make up your muscles are not used by the body to produce energy during fasting. It is incredibly inefficient and requires a lot of energy to exhaust muscles in the first place.

The energy you get by breaking down protein from your muscles does not provide more energy than carbohydrates. Also, it doesn't make sense that the body will destroy the functional tissues (our flesh) that we must use every day.

I Think It's Clear

Now think when our ancestors' hunters/gatherers did not have ready food. Could they hunt if their muscles were depleted for energy?

Not! Because it would make them weaker and slower. Accordingly, over time, more fragile and more time-consuming people would not be able to hunt and get food for the tribe just as effectively. The survival of our species during times of food shortages is due to our ability to use our fat stores as energy when there was a temporary shortage of food.

Therefore, it is entirely misleading to think that our muscles will be the first, and they will contract in a hungry state.

Here Is What Happens:

As the primary source of fuel for their needs during the first 24–48 hours without food. Your body will use sugar (in the body; it is stored as glycogen). After 48 hours, your body will begin to open and gain access to your fat reserves as an energy source.

This means that it will begin to break down the fat stored in the body for fuel as soon as sugar (glycogen) is depleted. The average person in the body has between 50,000 and 100,000 calories of fat. This is equivalent to accumulated fat for almost a month.

During a period of short-term fasting, exhaustion and breakdown of muscles do not occur.

Myth 3: Starvation Puts the Body in a "Malnutrition Mode"

In a hungry state, the body does not receive new food, which causes a calorie deficit. However, this caused some fears that starvation would lead to exhaustion. The loss of essential vitamins and minerals and, as a rule, will make us weak and depleted. Fasting lasts less than 24 hours (often called periodic fasting). Therefore, there is no need to worry about a lack of vitamins or minerals.

Mainly because we make up for everything that was lost with the food we eat on the same day. With prolonged fasting for 24 hours or longer, I always recommend adding sodium, potassium, and magnesium.

This is because, in a state of starvation, your kidneys coincide with a drop in insulin levels. Release the excess water we hold. And they remove together with excess water these vital trace elements that we need for cellular function. Keep in mind that this is not enough for malnutrition.

Malnutrition Supplement:

When people think of malnutrition, they think of poor, hungry children in Africa with bloated bellies. With sunken eyes with thin arms and legs. Remember, this does not happen during fasting.

However, the big food companies want you to believe that this will happen if you skip a meal. And why not? If you eat all the time, you consume their foods. The only thing that bothers them in this scenario is their profit.

Congratulations that you have come so far in my botanical safari, and that you're on approximately 1/2 WAY.

Myth 4: Low Blood Sugar

Here, many people are bewildered and confused. For those of us who do not have type 1 diabetes and are receiving medication for it, we may experience pseudo-symptoms of hypoglycemia.

True hypoglycemia is for patients with type 1 diabetes, and even then, it is usually the result of taking the drugs they take. For the rest of us, insulin resistance, low glycogen levels, and cortisol are common culprits disguised as hypoglycemia.

All Have Similar Symptoms with Low Blood Sugar

Ironically, things like insulin resistance, glycogen levels, and cortisol can be improved by fasting. When you are hungry, you are not taking any new sugar. Combine this with the fact that the brain and other organs require a small amount of sugar for a healthy metabolism. Beginners may experience things like trembling, headaches, and muscle weakness.

The answer is NO, I repeat. DO NOT eat anything sweet at this time.

It does not make sense to feed the system quick sugar if you have insulin resistance. Higher blood insulin or low glycogen stores. It's like giving an alcoholic some alcohol to make him feel better for a while!

To Solve This Problem, It Makes No Sense to Feed the Body with Sugar

People who experience symptoms of low blood sugar. They may try supplements with magnesium, potassium, and sodium. Vitamins and mineral supplements can help prevent nutrient deficiencies and stop shivering, headaches, and muscle weakness.

And here is a super cool, little-known fact - your body can make its sugar when it is hungry! Gluconeogenesis is a process in which the body produces its sugar.

Myth 5 - When I Eat Again, Food Turns into Fat!

When you decide to disrupt your fasting, your body will seek to replenish glycogen stores in the liver and muscles. We usually store about 2,000 calories in the liver, and it is the most natural source of energy for the body to access and use.

Thus, being a tremendously efficient machine for your body, he will probably want to replenish his most straightforward food source first. Only when your glycogen stores are full will your body begin sending excess calories to fat cells for storage.

Myth 6: The Most Important Meal of the Day Is Breakfast

We were told again and again that we should eat almost immediately after our awakening. The right breakfast is the right day off. The truth is that we were hungry while sleeping. And this is entirely normal. You need to eat then only when you feel hunger. Not only because you woke up, but also because you are hungry.

When you wake up, drink a glass of water - most likely, your hunger will disappear. Feelings of hunger and thirst are almost identical. You will probably find that your desire is masked by thirst.

The most important meal is when it is time to eat according to your fasting schedule. If you do short daily fasts, this is usually around lunch.

Myth 7: When Fasting, You Need to Change Your Lifestyle

There are many holidays in our life - Christmas, Birthdays, Weddings, Just meeting friends in nature, and this is entirely normal.

Good food must be shared with the people we love. And the essential events that accompany this. The beauty of intermittent fasting is that it has the right fasting scheme. Fasting fits perfectly into all the vital facts in your life. So, this is just a matter of choice and habit.

What the supporters of starvation myths mostly forget. So, this is about the health benefits of fasting.

Intermittent Fasting Protocols

Feedback and Orientation about My Interval Fasting Success

I've always been a friend of documentation! For thirty years, I have kept diaries and logs of various kinds: training diaries, nutrition diaries, transformation logs, and records of my challenges.

These labels give me feedback and enable —scientific work.‖ It is also fun and allows me to keep a precise overview. You quickly forget what you tried a few weeks, months, and years ago.

Through regular records, I have the opportunity to look back, what has led to success and what has led to a dead end. I show you how I document my interval fasting and clearly.

The Most Common Fasting Protocols

Since fasting is a waiver of food, bedtime is a part of fasting. So, each of us fasts for a few hours anyway during sleep. It is not without reason that breakfast is called the first meal after slumber, in English breakfast, i.e., ―break the fast‖ or translated into German ―fasting break.‖ Depending on the goal you are pursuing, different protocols and approaches to intermittent fasting are appropriate.

- Alternation of posts: This type of food involves fasting every other day. On fasting days, you can opt-out of eating altogether or limit your intake to 500 calories per day. On non-hungry days, you should follow a healthy keta diet as usual.

- 16/8 Post: The 16/8 alternating ketosis plan consists of fasting for 16 hours a day and restricting food intake to 8 hours a day. This usually means that you don't have to eat anything after dinner and skip breakfast the next morning.

- Diet 5: 2: In this plan, you follow a standard keta diet for five days a week and limit your intake to 500-600 calories for the remaining two days.

- 23/1 Kato Intermittent Fasting: Using this intermittent fasting method, you should restrict your meals to only one hour per day and fast for the remaining 23 hours of the day.

The List for Interval Fasting

Most of the time, I keep such logs and lists for three weeks. This provides a good overview of my daily behavior and shows how changing the individual parameters works. This is how you can see whether a certain period of fasting helps you lose weight, burn fat, build muscle or to understand which form of intermittent fasting best gives you what gives you the most energy and well-being:

Example week: week 1/3, day 1-7 / 21

Monday:

83.3 kg

18 hours of fasting,

1ST meal at noon, last meal at 6 p.m.

6 hours meal window

Eaten: 2 shakes, one salad, one sizeable main meal

Tuesday:

83.0 kg

Fasting for 20 hours

1ST meal at 2 p.m., the last lunch at 7 p.m.

5 hours meal window

Little hunger, one shake, 1 gr. the main meal, yogurt

Wednesday:

83 kg

17 hours of fasting,

1ST meal at noon, the last lunch at 7 p.m.

7 hours meal window

Very hungry, no-nails training, then two shakes, two large meals

Thursday:

82.8 kg

18 hours of fasting,

1ST meal at 1 p.m., the last lunch at 6 p.m.

5 hours meal window

Only raw food: smoothie, salad, sprouts + fruit

Friday:

82.6 kg

18 hours of fasting,

1ST meal at noon, the last lunch at 8 p.m.

Very hungry → longer meal windows (8 hours)

Saturday:

82.5 kg

16 hours of fasting,

1ST meal at noon, the last lunch at 8 p.m.

Stopped too late, high carb, flatulence

8-hour meal window

Sunday:

83.4 kg

16 hours of fasting,

1ST meal at noon, last meal at 6 p.m.

6 hours meal window

Perfect! 2 shakes, high protein, glycogen stores full of yesterday

Conclusion

That's what it looks like to me. You can also expand your list and write down exactly what you ate every day, whether you trained, what type of training you do on which day (although I keep a training diary, which I can highly recommend!), Including you feel what digestion, quality of sleep, detoxification, etc. are like.

Also, whether you eat low carb, high carb, high protein, high fat, little fat, raw food, or vegan, or whether you test dietary supplements, you can add all of this to your interval fasting list.

Draw the list on a piece of paper or create it on the PC and print it out, hang it on the fridge and off you go!

This gives you an overview of which form of interval fasting has led to which results for you at what time. This is suitable for almost all goals, such as fat burning and weight loss, muscle building and weight gain, detox and detoxification, food intolerance, and much more.

Alternate Day Fasting

The Basics of Alternate Day Fasting

Alternate Day Fasting extends the basic idea of interval fasting. Instead of dividing individual hours, the whole day becomes an interval summarized and determined either as a —fasting day‖ or an —eating day.‖ With Alternate Day Fasting, you alternate with your diet - fasting on one day and eating frequently again the next.

In this context, —fasting‖ means that you should consume as few calories as possible on fasting days. Usually, the plans recommend a maximum of 500 calories, which is about a quarter of your daily calorie needs. On this page, you can calculate your exact daily calorie needs by entering your age, weight, gender, and healthy activities.

On the dining days, however, you can eat as you please, just as your body was used to before starting the diet.

The Top 5 Scientifically-Based Benefits of Alternate Day Fasting

More and more scientific studies are proving the effects of Alternate Day Fasting on weight loss, reducing the risk of heart disease, and improving fat and blood sugar levels.

Interestingly, a case study even supports the thesis that interval fasting in general and alternate-day fasting, in particular, can reduce the symptoms of type 2 diabetes. Although it would be a bit premature to speak of healing powers here, various health benefits of ADF have already been proven.

This includes:

1. Lose Weight with Alternate Day Fasting

The experts agree that Alternate Day Fasting is excellent for losing weight. The background of the diet is simple enough.

Obesity has become a global epidemic in recent decades, the effects of which are still underestimated. The World Health Organization recently announced that the overweight population has almost tripled since 1975, an alarming increase. So, if you're struggling with weight problems, you should seriously consider changing your diet. Alternate Day Fasting can help you on your way.

A study published in the Nutrition Journal in 2013 found that after just 12 weeks of Alternate Day Fasting, an average decrease in fat mass of almost 4 kg was found. In addition to these results, a separate, recent study found that alternate-day fasting tended to make people aged 50 to 59 lose weight faster than participants in other age groups.

Extreme weight loss can then be recorded when Alternate Day Fasting is associated with endurance exercises, such as a study from 2013 suggests that was published in journal Obesity. By combining exercise and fasting, you can burn at least twice as much fat.

2. A Healthy Heart

Heart disease is the biggest reason for death as the whole world. It is estimated that cardiac and vascular diseases made more than one worldwide in 2016. Third of all deaths - and yet only a few people prevent this suffering. Alternate day fasting helps in many ways to reduce the risk of heart disease. The diet:

- **Promotes weight loss.**
- **Cleans the blood of bad cholesterol (LDL).**
- **Increases the level of good cholesterol (HDL).**
- **It lowers high blood pressure.**
- **Minimizes the generation of harmful fats (triglycerides).**

3. Checking Blood Sugar

A high blood sugar level occurs when the body does not produce enough insulin or does not use the available insulin properly (insulin resistance). If the blood sugar level remains too high for a long time, the person affected can develop diabetes.

Studies have shown that alternate day fasting, as well as other forms of interval fasting, help to lower blood sugar. The change in diet works by reducing insulin in the blood while increasing sensitivity to it.

4. Alternate Day Fasting Promotes Autophagy

Both long-term and short-term fasting triggers the process of autophagy in the body, in which unused, damaged, and potentially harmful cell components are recycled. Put, autophagy is the body's process of removing unwanted substances from cells.

This process, in turn, reduces the risk of an outbreak for numerous diseases. These include infections, heart disease, obesity, or even cancer.

5. Alternate Day Fasting as a Fountain of Youth

The limitation of the total calorie intake, which is achieved by the Alternate Day Fasting, has been shown in many animal experiments as a way to significantly extend your life.

In these studies, animals that received all the necessary nutrients but fewer calories lived longer than those who received more calories. This variance in lifespan manifests itself primarily in a significantly lower risk of being affected by age-related diseases.

One study, in particular, found that a variant of Alternate Day Fasting increased the lifespan in male mice by primarily doing that

Cancer incidence has been delayed. However, these results should be used with caution as animal experiments do not meet the same requirements as human studies. A trend can still be seen.

Is Alternate Day Fasting Safe? Identify Potential Risks

It can be said that alternate-day fasting is an extremely safe method, mainly if the changeover is only carried out for a short time and is dealt with the appropriate knowledge. Long-term negative consequences for health have so far not been documented or have only been insufficiently documented.

As with most other diets, you are changing the diet can cause problems for people with chronic diseases such as high blood pressure or diabetes. If you suffer from a severe illness or take medication regularly, you should consult a doctor in advance before you start fasting.

Likewise, pregnant women, women who are breastfeeding, children, and underweight, should only draw up a fasting schedule when a doctor has given the green light for it.

If you are starting Alternate Day Fasting, you should be prepared for the following side effects:

- **Constipation**
- **Giddiness**
- **A general feeling of weakness**
- **Bad breath**
- **Sleep disorders**
- **Menstrual cycle irritation**
- **Mood swings, anxiety, and depressive symptoms in healthy people**

Fortunately, these problems don't occur often, and if they do, they only occur in a mild form. An intervention in the routines of the body also causes reactions to it.

Advantages:

With this method, significant calorie deficits of 3000-6000 kcal per week can be achieved. Bodyweight can be reduced quickly, especially at the start of a diet, and contribute to motivation to stay with it.

Disadvantages:

It is not entirely clear whether the health benefits that intermittent fasting brings also work with this method since people eat every day, and there is no longer a long time without calorie intake. In any case, weight loss and the reduction of body fat are clearly in the foreground

Conclusion

Alternate Day Fasting proves to be an effective way to lose weight. Various studies confirm the positive influence of the change in diet on the general state of health, especially if the fasting is only brief. The risk of heart disease has been proven to be reduced, and glucose metabolism improved.

Both standard and overweight (or obese) people can benefit from the benefits of Alternate Day Fasting. Many experts classify the diet as harmless if there are no other health problems. In comparison, ADF is a relatively safe method of fasting.

However, pregnant and breastfeeding women, underweight people, and minors should consult a doctor before starting the fasting program. The same applies if you are taking medication for high blood pressure or diabetes.

If you want to get on board fully and achieve optimal results, you should contact experts who will provide you with specific fasting plans.

The 16/8 Methods

Where Does 16: 8 Interval Fasting Come From?

Phases of fasting are nothing new to our bodies. In earlier times, it was typical for our ancestors that in times of deficiency, the stomach remained empty for hours or even days. As soon as the food was available, the reserves were filled up extensively.

The body usually survives small periods of hunger without any problems by storing energy reserves in various organs and tissues. If necessary, he can then use it.

Why Do You Have to Take Breaks Between Meals?

The 16-hour break of fasting gives the body a break. During this time, the metabolism can be brought back to normal, toxins that have accumulated in the liver can be better excreted, and the body can process insulin better again.

Ideally, the body can switch back and forth between sugar and fat metabolism better, which improves fat metabolism.

Can You Lose Weight with Interval Fasting 16: 8?

Interval fasting is not a typical diet. So, whether you lose weight or not depends on the individual. If you pay attention to eating as healthy and low-calorie as possible during the eight hours, weight reduction can be achieved.

Of course, you can also sin, for example, and have a pizza, as long as you make the other meals a little smaller. It is essential to keep the total number of calories during the meal phase lower than usual. A gentle reduction in calorie intake of around 20 percent of the typical daily requirement is usually recommended. In the case of an adult woman, that would be about 1400 - 1600 kilocalories per day, which can be consumed if one assumes a daily requirement of 1800 - 2000 kilocalories.

How Does A 16: 8 Interval Fasting Work?

In addition to weight loss, 16: 8 intervals, fasting has many other health-improving effects. It is generally assumed that fasting has a positive impact on healtH1.

The pauses between food intakes stimulate cell cleaning (autophagy) 2. That means the body can clean up and detoxify the cells. This has a positive effect on blood sugar levels3, which can prevent diabetes risk. Blood pressure and cholesterol levels can also be regulated.

In contrast to longer fasting cures or so-called crash diets, the metabolism is also not throttled, and the muscle mass is not reduced. This reduces the risk of a yo-yo effect after the end of the fasting cure. Even the body only begins to lose muscle mass after a fasting period of around 48 hours.

How Does Interval Fasting Work: The 16: 8 Instructions?

The focus of interval fasting is the precise delimitation of the fasting and eating phase. Food is consumed for a limited time for 8 hours a day, the remaining 16 hours fast. Everything else can be designed relatively individually. That means when and what you eat during the 8 hours, everyone can decide for themselves.

It is recommended to take two meals. Breakfast or dinner is omitted at will. Then you have to do without food for 16 hours at a time.

Intermittent Fasting: Learn to Do Without Food for 16 Hours

Lent of 16 hours may not be that easy at first for some people. If you have problems giving up food for so long, you can first fast for 12 or 14 hours and then gradually increase.

Over time, the body will get used to the new rhythm. It can also help to get the hunger holes filled with thin vegetable broth and unsweetened teas, to begin with. During breaks, the body can also use its energy reserves and stimulate fat burning.

Which Drinks And Foods Are Particularly Suitable For 16: 8 Interval Fasting?

Especially if you want to reduce your weight, the following foods and drinks are suitable:

- **Lots of fresh fruits and vegetables**
- **Nuts and dried fruit as a snack instead of cookies and chips**
- **Protein and fiber-rich foods**
- **Silent Waters**
- **Unsweetened teas**
- **Black, unsweetened coffee**
- **Superfoods such as chia seeds**

Which Drinks and Foods Should Be Avoided With 16: 8 Interval Fasting?

The following should be avoided during the fasting phase:

- **Any food intake**
- **Drinks containing sugar and calories**
- **Juices**

In principle, everything can be consumed during the meal phase, but it is advisable to do without the following things:

- **Greasy foods**
- **Sugar and candy**
- **Processed carbohydrates such as white bread.**

How Much Can You Lose In 16: 8 Interval Fasting?

Everybody responds differently to a diet and how much you ultimately lose depends on different things. On the one hand, how much overweight you were at the start of the fasting cure, because the more body fat you have, the more the body can naturally lose weight.

On the other hand, weight loss depends on how you eat during this time and how much sport you also do during the time.

Unsuccessful 16: 8 Interval Fasting: Why Don't I Lose Weight?

If you do not lose weight despite the fasting phases, it may be because you overeat in the eating phases. Because if you eat more than your body consumes, you negate the benefits of fasting.

Another reason can be the choice of food. If you only eat unhealthy, high-calorie, and sugary food during the 8 hours, you cannot hope for weight loss success. Only in connection with a healthy diet can 16: 8 fasting lead to weight loss.

The Advantages and Disadvantages of 16: 8 Interval Fasting

Overall, this fasting method has fewer disadvantages than other diets and weight loss trends. Here you will find an overview of all the advantages and disadvantages.

What Are the Advantages Of 16: 8 Interval Fasting?

• You can lose weight gently and maintain your body weight in the long term

- **Improvement in cholesterol levels**
- **Diabetes can be improved**
- **Improved sugar and fat metabolism**
- **No cravings or feelings of weakness**
- **The diet is suitable for everyday use**
- **The yo-yo effect can be avoided**
- **No muscle mass is lost in the body**

What are the disadvantages of 16: 8 intervals fasting?

- **Strong feelings of hunger can occur, especially in the transition phase**
- **Some people suffer from food cravings as a result**

- **16 hours without food is not for everyone**
- **Fasting alone is usually not expected to be successful in losing weight**

For Whom Is 16: 8 Interval Fasting Suitable?

The fasting method is suitable for everyone who wants to reduce body fat without having to restrict themselves too much when eating. Or also for people who would like to maintain their body weight without having to do without feasting.

It is also suitable for all forms of nutrition, from vegan to all-eater.

Most will find it easier to give up food for only 16 hours than to go through an entire diet or fasting regimen. The 16: 8 cycle is also suitable for sporty people. You can incorporate the sports program into the fasting phase in the morning and then replenish your energy reserves at noon and in the evening.

The 5/2 Method

The Secret of the 5: 2 Interval Fasting Method

The results of the 5: 2 diet, which is becoming increasingly popular worldwide, are astonishing: the kilos are falling, and health is improving. You don't have to keep dieting all the time, eat significantly less than usual two days a week. You can continue to eat as usual on the remaining five days of the week. That sounds good.

But what is really behind the 5: 2 method? How does it work? Who is it suitable for? Can you lose weight with this interval fasting method? And how does The Fast Diet, as the 5: 2 diet, is called, compare to other forms of intermittent fasting? We'll tell you.

How Does The 5: 2 diet Work?

With the 5: 2 diet, a variant of interval fasting, you usually eat five days a week and significantly less on two days a week. Women are allowed to eat 500 calories and men 600 calories on the two days of fasting.

The easiest way to get the 5: 2 diet to work is not to put the two days of fasting directly behind one another, but, e.g., B. fasts on Mondays and Thursdays or Tuesdays and Fridays. Instead of eating the allowed calories of 500 or 600 calories at once, it should be more convenient to split them into two meals. Then you could have a small breakfast and a small dinner on the two fasting days.

So, you can drink a glass of buttermilk and eat two boiled eggs with some smoked salmon in the evening. Or eat a piece of fruit with some yogurt in the morning and a small salad with some steamed vegetables in the evening.

The inventors of the diet recommend eating high-fiber and high-protein foods on fasting days and avoiding quickly digestible carbohydrates. You should drink enough on the fasting days, but only calorie-free drinks such as water, tea, or black coffee.

Interestingly, the participants do not eat more than usual on regular eating days. Therefore, the 5: 2 diet saves a lot of calories in the long run. This will decrease, and that is healthy.

However, this is not a diet in the conventional sense, but a nutritional concept that you can permanently integrate into your everyday life.

The Advantages of the 5: 2 Diet:

The 5: 2 method does not require any complicated rules and is easy to implement.

There are no permanent bans or restrictions on the Fast Diet. This is psychologically beneficial and can help contain cravings. Through regular fasting days, the weight drops and unnecessary pounds are lost.

Severe calorie restriction has positive health effects. The insulin sensitivity of the cells and the blood values improve.

Because you only limit your calorie intake for two days but otherwise usually eat, your metabolism remains active and does not fall asleep like with conventional diets. This protects against the infamous yo-yo effect.

The 5: 2 diet is a permanently viable strategy for a healthy, long life and not a conventional time-limited diet.

The Disadvantages of the 5: 2 Diet:

The strict adherence to the calorie restriction on the fasting days with the 5: 2 method is very complicated and complicated. It takes proper planning and preparation to limit your calories in this way. You have to find new recipes that match and adhere to them correctly.

Exceptions are not allowed on the fasting days. Spontaneous dinners with friends or just having a cappuccino are canceled these days. The fasting days, therefore, need to be well planned and allow little social flexibility.

The low number of calories can lead to headaches and reduced performance on fasting days. The feeling of hunger can also get very strong at the beginning. However, these symptoms usually go away after a while if you follow the 5: 2 diet regularly.

The 5: 2 Diet: What Science Says

A new study on the 5: 2 method led Dr. Michelle Larvie of the Genesis Breast Cancer Prevention Center in Manchester. It divided 115 women into three groups.

The women in the first group were put on a Mediterranean diet with only 1500 calories a day. The second group was supposed to eat only 650 calories two days a week by the 5: 2 food and was allowed to eat normally on the remaining days of the week. The women in the third group should avoid carbohydrates two days a week, but were allowed to eat without any calorie restriction.

The results were terrific.

After three months, the women on the two —two-day diets‖ lost almost 5 kg, nearly twice as much as the women in the first group, who had to count calories continuously. Insulin resistance had also improved significantly in groups two and three. With that came, Dr. Larvie concluded that calorie restriction only two days a week offers the same and possibly even more benefits than a healthy, full-time, low-calorie diet.

Why Is The 5: 2 Diet So Positive?

Our body and our genes were created under conditions of lack, interrupted by the occasional —big feast.‖ So, we are well adapted to phases without food.

And even if we find fasting uncomfortable at first, according to the principle of the Hermes's, what does no harm makes us stronger. While starving for too long is harmful, we benefit from shorter periods without food. That makes us healthier and more resilient.

For Whom Is The 5: 2 Diet Suitable?

The 5: 2 diet is suitable for anyone who wants to do something good for their health. The substantial calorie restriction two days a week has been shown to have a beneficial effect on health. The 5: 2 method can also help you lose weight. On average, you lose approximately 1 kg of weight per month with this variant of interval fasting. If you don't want to lose weight and keep your weight, you only have to fast one day a week instead of two. As simple as that.

Especially for people who cannot cope with the daily limitation of the meal window to 8, 6 or only 4 hours, as is familiar with other forms of classic intermittent fasting, the 5: 2 diet can be a sensible alternative to traditional interval fasting,

For Whom Is The 5: 2 Diet Not Suitable?

But the 5: 2 method is not suitable for everyone. Adolescents, breastfeeding, and pregnant women generally have an increased calorie requirement and should refrain from the 5: 2 diet. People with diseases, mainly if they, e.g., For example, if you are taking medication to lower blood pressure or regulate blood sugar, the 5: 2 diet, like any other form of intermittent fasting, should be discussed in advance with a doctor or therapist.

Our Conclusion on the 5: 2 Diet

In our eyes, the 5: 2 method is more of a diet than a form of intermittent fasting. Intermittent fasting is about extending the phases without food. The 5: 2 method, on the other hand, is about severely limiting the number of calories two days a week. That is a big difference! Eating a few calories has a different impact on the hormonal and metabolic levels than consuming no calories over some time.

In our eyes, it would make more sense to consume the permitted number of calories of 500 or 600 calories with the 5: 2 diet in one meal, to significantly extend the fasting phase. However, since we generally find calorie counting annoying, we would recommend the so-called one-meal-a-day method (OMAD) or the EatStopEat method (= IF 24/0). Here, too, you can eat once a day, but without paying attention to the number of calories. The successes that can be achieved with these forms of interval fasting are at least no less remarkable than with the 5: 2 diet.

In any case, it is easier for us not to eat for 16, 18, 20, or even 24 or 36 hours than to be satisfied with a mini portion. On the other hand, some people get along correctly with the 5: 2 method.

So once again: You can only find out whether the 5: 2 diet is for you by trying it out yourself. To benefit from the advantages of fasting, you should eat 500 or 600 calories in one meal rather than spread them over two meals.

The Warrior Diet (The 20 Hour Fast)

How 20: 4 Intermittent Fasting Works

With the Warrior Diet, the time window for daily food intake is reduced to 4 hours. In these four hours (this should be the evening hours), as much as is fed what the refrigerator has to offer. In the other 20 hours, there is no need to refrain from eating altogether. Just as the warrior sometimes paused while roaming the country, smaller amounts of dairy products (e.g., a mug of yogurt), fresh fruits and vegetables, and protein-rich snacks such as hard-boiled eggs and nuts can be consumed during the day. You should also drink plenty of low-calorie drinks such as water and tea.

Most people fast during the day and put the four-hour meal window in the early evening. But here, too, everyone has to find out for themselves which time window fits best. You can eat two meals or a more substantial dinner during this time. Others eat a first lunch around 12 or 1 p.m. and a more significant dinner around 5 p.m. before the time window closes. You have to decide for yourself which times in interval fasting work better for you. It is usually easier to avoid food during the day because you are distracted from work, sports, and other activities.

Being Active Does No Harm

Similar to the warriors who used to roam for hours to hunt animals, you should be as active as possible during the day with the Warrior Diet. Of course, this is not so easy if you have to spend the day at your desk. Nevertheless, try to do sports, for example during a lunch break or in the late afternoon before the four-hour window for eating. After eating, on the other hand, you should no longer exercise. The body comes to rest in the evening and then concentrates entirely on eating and digestion.

Even with 20: 4 intervals fasting, your food should always contain wholesome and protein-rich meals, i.e., you should mainly focus on meat, fish, eggs, vegetables, and fruit and only use carbohydrates sparingly. Here are the recipes on our site.

The Warrior Diet Brings These Health Benefits

Intermittent fasting has many health benefits, which also result from the Warrior Diet: This reduces the risk of inflammation, regulates blood sugar levels better, and strengthens the health of the brain. A long-term study even found that short-term fasting can lower the risk of Alzheimer's. However, this applies to all forms of short-term fasting. Here are more reasons why interval fasting is right for you too.

These Challenges Arise With 20: 4 Interval Fasting

In addition to the health benefits already described above, this diet does not only bring positive things.

Fasting For 20 Hours Is Not Always Easy

In our view, the most obvious challenge of the Warrior Diet is that you can only eat 4 hours a day. That may not be a problem on certain days. On other days, this is undoubtedly difficult. Our experience here is that the 20-hour fast is a significant hurdle in a healthy life and social activities, and it requires the right amount of self-discipline. An invitation to brunch or dinner together can be a challenge. Who wants to sit next to it and eat nothing?

Again, it is essential that you have to find out for yourself whether 20: 4 interval fasting suits you. Try it better at the start of interval fasting with the gentler 16: 8 method, and if you find that you can cope well with Lent, you can also try the tightened Warrior Diet. So, we did it, and it worked well. Nevertheless, we have to say quite frankly that the restriction was too big for us and we, therefore, prefer the more flexible 16 hours fast.

Some People Don't Tolerate the Warrior Diet So Well

Eating only 4 hours a day is a form of nutrition that not all people should follow. For the following groups of people, in particular, this should be viewed as critical:

- **Children**
- **People with eating disorders**
- **Pregnant or breastfeeding women**
- **Underweight people**
- **Athlete**
- **People with certain diseases (diabetes 1, heart problems or similar)**

In the last 20 hours of fasting has a not inconsiderable impact on human hormonal balance. This method is also considered critical for women. Since fasting can also affect the period, we recommend our article intermittent fasting in women for further reading.

If you want an overview of the types of interval fasting, follow this link for our simple interval fasting guide.

This Approach Can Lead to Eating Disorders

Let's be honest with ourselves. In the four hours of eating a day, we naturally want to eat enough. By eating so much, compared to the healthy eating rhythm, nutritionists warn of a negative effect on your eating habits. If you eat only such large portions, you can also lead to an eating disorder. It is, therefore, essential to question yourself critically and to keep a close eye on your eating habits.

Other Side Effects Have Also Been Observed

As with other changes, side effects can also occur with the Warrior Diet, including:

- **Laxity/lack of energy**
- **Low blood sugar**
- **Fatigue**
- **Slight dizziness**
- **Feelings of fear/anxiety**

- **Extremely hungry**
- **Hormonal imbalances**
- **Rapid irritability**

In our view, it is merely essential to listen to yourself and your body. If it doesn't go away, you should see a doctor or limit the periods in which you fast.

What Is the Best Way to Start the Warrior Diet?

There are two ways in which to start at 20: 4 intervals of fasting. We tried the first variant ourselves. We first started with the 16: 8 method, and only when we had a good feeling here was Lent extended to 20 hours.

A second variant is a recommendation from Hofmekler itself. He recommends starting the 20: 4 intervals fasting with different weeks with different eating focuses. The intention is to get the body used to use fat more quickly as an energy reserve:

The First Week (Also Called Detoxification Week)

You shouldn't eat much in the 20-hour window this week, but you shouldn't fast yet. You should eat vegetable juices, clear broths, and dairy products such as goat cheese.

In the 4 hours you eat a healthy salad with oil-vinegar dressing, for example. After that, you can have large or several smaller meals with vegetable proteins (e.g., beans) with smaller portions of cheese and cooked vegetables.

Tea, water and small amounts of milk may be drunk all the time

The Second Week (Also Called High-Fat Week)

You shouldn't eat much in the 20-hour window this week, but you shouldn't fast yet. Here you eat vegetable juices, clear meat broths, and dairy products like goat cheese.

In the 4 hours, you can also eat a healthy salad with oil and vinegar dressing. After that, you can eat large or several smaller meals with pure animal protein, cooked vegetables, and a handful of nuts.

Nothing is eaten this week with wheat or starchy foods (corn, beans, potatoes, etc.)

The Third Week (Cycle Week)

This week you switch between times with a high carbohydrate or high protein content.

A day or two with high carbohydrates. Then follow a day or two with a high protein and low carbohydrate content. Another day or two with high glucose. And again a day or two with a high protein and low carbohydrate content

When you're done with the three weeks, you can start over. In this way, the body learns faster how it can gain energy from fat reserves. A critical point here is that there are no portion sizes or calorie plans with the Warrior Diet.

It is up to you when you switch to the regular 20-hour fast rhythm. The important thing is that you feel comfortable in the approach, and your hunger attacks are no longer too strong.

What Can I Eat and Drink?

20: 4 intervals fasting allows you to drink low-calorie drinks such as water, (black) coffee and tea during the day, and even snack on small things like a handful of nuts, a piece of fruit, or a protein shake. Still, 20 hours is a very long time to fast. Supporters of this diet report that eating less food makes them feel more energetic and fitter during the day, as the body uses the non-food time for intermittent fasting to detoxify and burn fat.

Whether all of this is true is, of course, questionable. Who can say today whether the warriors of the early days did not take food supplies with them on the hunt or in between killed a small animal and consumed it during a more extended break? It is also clear that a physically active hunter, whose mind was focused on tracking, hunting and killing animals, wasted much less thought on the needs of the body than the modern desk warrior, who only worked with Excel spreadsheets and PowerPoint presentations wrestles and has mental idle again and again.

You can find more detailed help in the articles on −Intermittent fasting eat something‖   and −Intermittent fasting drinks something.‖

Our Conclusion About 20: 4 Interval Fasting

We tried the 20-hour fasting method. There are currently no explicit studies that dealt with this method alone. However, we assume that all of the positive effects of interval fasting also affect here. As with any interval fasting method, everyone has to find out for themselves which way is the most suitable.

The Eat Stop Eat Method

What Does "Eat-Stop-Eat" Mean?

–Eat-stop-eat‖ is a specific form of intermittent fasting, which, according to its inventor Brad Pylon, can effectively and sustainably lose weight with only one or two fasting units 24 hours a week and reduce your body fat percentage.

The basic concept is quickly explained: it is about fasting for one or two days a week (not more often!) For 24 hours (no longer!). So, you shouldn't consume any calories during this time. However, water, coffee (black), green tea, herbal tea, and even diet drinks and sweeteners are allowed in the fasting periods. You can continue to eat as usual on the remaining days.

Those who fast twice a week should take at least two eating days between the two days of fasting.

The trick is: if you fast for –only‖ 24 hours, you can eat every day. On a fasting day, for example, you stop eating after breakfast and then start breakfast the next day as usual. You can also fast from lunch to lunch or dinner for dinner.

Pylon, a graduate nutritionist and long-time employee of a nutritional supplement company in Toronto, is free to choose which rhythm to choose. The important thing is that once you have found the right rhythm for yourself, you stick with it.

Pylon recommends that you eat a sufficient amount of fruits and vegetables, but since it does not see its concept as a conventional diet, it does not want to ban food generally. So what tastes is allowed.

Also, the intermittent fasting expert recommends doing muscle training at least twice a week so that no muscle mass is lost during fasting.

With each 24-hour fast, it should be possible to lose between 1.5 to 3 pounds (which corresponds to approximately 0.65 to 1.3 kg) of weight (not pure fat!). The heavier the person and the higher their body fat percentage, the greater the weight loss.

Pylon needs to emphasize that his –eat-stop-eat‖ concept is not a temporary and, therefore, temporary measure, but a lifestyle that should become a habit.

Eat-Stop-Eat: Does This Form of Intermittent Fasting Do What It Promises?

Anyone who has been reading here for a long time knows that both Jens and I are big fans of intermittent fasting. We have been practicing different forms of short-term fasting for several years and are very enthusiastic. You can find out more about my experience here >> we have not yet tested the –Eat-Stop-Eat‖ variant, but the theory behind it sounds convincing.

Pylon differentiates between two different metabolic states, which from his point of view, are opposed to each other like Yin and Yang. Either our body is in the state of being built (–feeding‖) or in the state of being broken down (–almost‖). You cannot do both at the same time.

In the state of construction, our body draws its energy from the nutrients from the last meal. When dismantled, it consumes them from its storage. To put it: when we are set up, we become thicker, and when we are dismantled, we become thinner.

As long as these phases alternate and are on an equal footing, we keep our weight. If they get out of balance, we increase or decrease.

Pylon regards the fact that we are eating almost always as the most significant major evil of our diet today. Snacks and snacks for the three main meals are the rules, not the exception. Only when we are asleep, do we give our body a break of a few hours.

So, we are almost continuously in the state of –feeding.‖ As a result, the relationship between assembly and disassembly is out of balance. A conclusion is an increasing number of people struggling with obesity.

Why 24 Hours?

Pylon, who had to evaluate all the fat burning and muscle building studies for his job for many years, found in all of his research that short-term fasting breaks of up to 48 hours, unlike longer-lasting fasting periods of 72 hours or more, have no adverse effects.

With such short periods of fasting, no muscles are broken down, the metabolism is not reduced, and therefore no yo-yo effect is triggered. No hormonal disturbances are to be expected, either. On the contrary, short-term fasting has numerous health benefits, at least that has been shown by multiple studies on humans and animals, which the author lists in his book.

The Advantages of Intermittent Fasting (IF) / Short-Term Fasting:

- Short-term fasting lowers insulin levels and increases insulin sensitivity. This primarily prevents diabetes and the associated consequential damage.

- Intermittent fasting lowers blood sugar, preventing excess weight, increased blood lipid levels, and premature aging.

- It increases the body's ability to use energy from the stored fat reserves and thus boosts fat burning.

- Intermittent fasting increases HGH release, a hormone that is involved in fat loss, muscle building, and rejuvenation.

- IF also lowers the rate of inflammation in the body

- Stimulates the cleansing and renewal of cells, the so-called autophagy, or auto phagocytosis.

What Is the Right and Healthy Way to Fast

Why Fasting Is So Healthy

Fasting is much more than not eating. Researchers are amazed to see the powerful effects of systematically doing without our bodies. And how beneficial it is on the course of diseases. An interview with Dr. Hanie Luck, biochemist, and author of the GEO cover story —The Healing Power of Fasting.‖

Fasting - Isn't That Against Nature, Where We Have to Eat To Stay Productive To Survive?

Until my research, I felt similar. Fast? A painful procedure for slimming fanatics or anti-pleasure ascetics. That's what I thought when I was told not to eat. No wonder. Growing up in a family where everything took place around the richly laid the table, on which there was always something good - cooked and seasoned with conversation, enjoyment, and community. Fasting is just as much a part of nature as eating. Animals and people of all cultures do it, wanted, and unwanted. It is a beneficial principle in terms of evolutionary biology. It has always helped us to survive hunger times efficiently for hunting and gathering - and it triggers healing processes in the body.

How Can Fasting Contribute to Our Health?

The voluntary food withdrawal is not only rejuvenating and regenerating. The medical significance is also becoming increasingly apparent. Because of fasting acts like a - wholesome - shock on the body. He turns physiology upside down and triggers entire cascades of biochemical reactions. For example, unique cleaning mechanisms are stimulated: the garbage disposal and the recycling system of the cells. Or: Fasting has been shown to inhibit inflammation and lower high blood pressure. Or: As the latest research shows, fasting can even help people with cancer.

Fasting Has Always Been Done. Why Is the Topic Only Now Being Recognized By Science?

Because the findings in fasting research are going through the roof, research into the fantastic molecular waste disposal of the body now even makes the concept of —slags,‖ which has been rejected for so long, appear in a new light. Even more important are the results of great new experiments, which show, for example, that fasting and age genes and cancer genes in the genome are immobilized. And very important: Scientists are exploring new, simple types of fasting for everyone.

What Is the Difference Between Fasting and Diet?

In contrast to diets, fasting is not just about losing weight, but primarily about detoxification, excretion, and regeneration. Also: The physiological difference between preceding food and dieting is excellent: When fasting, the body quickly switches to burning fat. In the end, no more prolonged sugar, but so-called ketones are used as an energy source. This unique —fasting metabolism‖ has positive effects on neurogenesis, the regeneration of brain cells. It is doubtful whether and when this happens on different diets.

Next: Diets always include the risk of malnutrition because you can't listen to your body (a diet usually prohibits certain foods), and the craving for something often means that the agency —translates‖ a deficiency into appetite. With fasting, you can eat whatever you want - unless you are fasting.

Chapter 2:
Benefits of Intermittent Fasting
for Women Over 50

Intermittent fasting is all the rage. Some of you might even consider it a fad. We certainly believe it has some incredible health and weight loss benefits. We talk about the pros and cons and a gentler and kinder approach to intermittent fasting. I have been coaching women for decades in the area of weight loss and health, and we are what you would consider mature women on 50. There are so many great health benefits to intermittent fasting like: -

- **Improved brain function**
- **Weight loss**
- **Fat burning of course**
- **Increased metabolism**
- **Anti-aging benefits**

There're so many benefits there are some downsides, especially for women in our age range, and why would you know we've mentioned at the beginning that this seems like a fad. The truth is it's healthy, and we wanted to become your new neural if you thought back 200 years ago the average woman lived on a farm. She got up the crack of dawn and went to bed right about sunset, and she probably only ate about maybe 11 or 12 hours a day tied her first meal at 9:00 maybe stopped eating at 6 or 7 p.m.

She was naturally fasting, and she was getting some of the health benefits. Of course, the weight loss benefits shade a lot more calories. So, that what we're asking you to start with and consider is what was a healthy normal in days past Robin was mentioning there are some downsides that we want to talk about before we tell you ours.

Gentler Kinder Approach to Fasting

That we think will work exceptionally well for mature women well one thing to look out for is to not necessarily jump into a long intermittent fast especially for women that are in our age bracket some of us have what's called

Adrenal Fatigue

You may or may not know if you have adrenal fatigue. If you have gotten a cortisol test, it will let you know, so we do recommend doing that there are some signs and symptoms to look for. There's a ton of them we're not going to go through all of them. Still, if you're super tired when you wake up in the morning you should start dragging yourself out of bed are you craving salty foods if you're gaining weight in the midsection is a sign of adrenal fatigue. The reason we bring this up is that if you do have that fasting, it puts stress on your body.

It's good stress for most people. Still, if you have adrenal fatigue, it can be a little detrimental, and it can cause your adrenal fatigue to get worse, and what we don't want to see happen as you go into adrenal burnout where you have zapped energy completely. So, there are some ways to prevent this

The Ageless Eating Cycle

It's going to be an element in our new book that's coming out, so I'm going to share today precisely what that is three steps to make this kinder and gentler for your body to make sure you're not putting undue stress

Step 1

You're ideally going to make it a goal to stop eating three hours before you go to bed at night that alone without even adding any other fasting can cut out so many excess calories and carbohydrates. So, forth then it's just a great practice yeah, every once in a while, you will eat your up for a special occasion or whatever but if you could make this your habit, you're going to have so many great benefits

Step 2

It would be to set a goal to make it a goal to fast for 12 hours every single day now that would mean if you have your last fight and food at 7 p.m. Then you wouldn't eat again until after seven days. But it's not that yummy baby or 8 p.m. and don't eat again until after 8:00. Now you have to listen to your body in making this goal. You may not be used to this. You might have a little bit of low blood sugar, and maybe you're able to make it 11 hours.

You can work your way up to 12 and let me say that if you do feel like you're, we call it balking at 10 hours or 11 hours. Because your body not adapted yet, you know what has a small snack at 10 hours or 11:00 or is that something a hundred fifty calories and then continue to fast for the next couple hours until you're ready to break it truly. You may have broken your fast, but it just gets you in that habit of moving towards that 12-hour goal.

I want you to know another fantastic benefit studies have shown that women who had breast cancer the reoccurrence rate of **breast cancer goes down significantly for women in fast 13 hours a day** on an average basis so that 12 to 13-hour mark has some other potential benefits shifting you from primary glucose burning to more fat burning.

Step 3

Go to the next level where intermittent fasting really kicks in and notches up some of the extra benefits again ketone production fat burning higher energy all of those do tend to increase as fast increases. But we'd like to see you move from that 12 hours to maybe 13, 14, And 15 and to cap out for most of you not all. But for most of you in about 16 hours so that would be 16 hours of fasting 8 hours of eating. I tend to be a little bit later eater and not eat again until noon. It's not that hard. We'll talk a bit of more how to gauge if it works for you, and I want to clarify that so if you're working towards 16 hours fast, not necessarily 16 hours every single day maybe three days a week maybe four days a week.

When you are working towards that longer fast, you maybe 16 hours one day. The next thing you might be back to 12 hours the next day you might be at 15, the next thing you might get 13 don't get hung up on the numbers and the hours. Listen to your body because your body is going to be telling you if you are getting a massive headache, you know what it's time to break that past even if your goal is for 16 hours 14 hours is okay. By the way, one significant caution there's a few of you that will do what's called **rebound heating you fast.**

You're doing great, and then all of a sudden, you can throw caution the wind. It's like oh, I thought that I could eat anything I want no this is a technique to help you hopefully miss that extra meal or so and not make up the calories on the other. We're in that in our eating window, and you're eating twice as much as you usually would if you like a little bit of support in the area of your nutrition and healthy weight loss we encourage.

Most Common Mistakes of Intermittent Fasting and How to Fix Them

Impossible to escape what seems to some to be a fashion effect. Everyone talks about intermittent fasting. I'm not going to make yet another copy of the hundreds of books already existing on the subject that only list the main benefits of intermittent fasting. If you have just come out of several years of hibernation and are still ignorant about it, a simple search on Google will fill all your gaps.

In this book, I especially want to talk to you about three big mistakes that seem to me to be recurring and which perhaps prevent you, too, from riding the wave of –fasting‖ ... and burning fat without needing to snack all the 2 hours. Intermittent fasting is an art.

Mistake Number 1: Abusing Stimulants (Coffee, Tea, Etc.)

In the world of intermittent fasting, it is generally accepted that you can eat or drink whatever you want as long as the food or drink contains no calories. Indeed, the goal of the fasting phase is to keep your insulin low to maintain the fat-burning mode. We know that lipids stimulate **a little**, proteins **moderately**, and carbohydrates a **lot** of insulin.

Remember: when the **insulin is high**, your body is in **storage** mode; when **insulin is low**, your body is in a **destocking** mode (fat burning).

If we stop there, any drink containing no calories is eligible for the fasting phase: tea, coffee, drinks containing false sugars. Stimulating drinks are also often recommended by several promoters of intermittent fasting. Caffeine is indeed well known in the world of fitness and food supplements to suppress appetite and speed up metabolism (with the key a potential bonus in terms of fat loss. at least in theory).

I have absolutely nothing against coffee lovers, having myself been a chronic drinker a few years ago. Still, we know very well that as a psychotropic drug, caffeine is nothing but doping legal. The fact that its consumption is culturally accepted does not change the fact that it is antinomy to fasting (intermittent or not) in terms of health.

The Harmful Effects of Caffeine in the Long Term

To understand this, let's already briefly summarize the action of caffeine on the body. Caffeine will take the place of a neuromodulator, adenosine, which usually has the role of slowing down nervous activity if necessary (energy deficit) while stimulating the action of the adrenal glands (production of adrenaline). In other words, coffee, and tea to a lesser extent, will produce a peak of energy by preventing the signal of fatigue from playing its role. A message which is not there to annoy us but rather to protect our potentially significant damage to the body, which could occur as a result of over-activity in the nervous system.

Coffee, a popular but not harmless drink for our health.

Concretely, when a person's nervous system begins to exhaust itself for various reasons (chronic lack of sleep or overwork, for example), the short-term –beneficial‖ effects of caffeine will be more and more felt. The person then becomes addicted to his little daily shoot and may start to multiply the cups during the day. After a few years of overwork, the person is so exhausted that he begins to manifest symptoms of caffeine intolerance more and more marked:

- **Tachycardia**
- **Nervousness**
- **Mood swings**
- **Intestinal disorders**
- **Cravings**

If you are in the latter case, the consumption of caffeine will cause stress such that your hormonal system will cause an increase in blood sugar (and therefore insulin), most of the time by going to draw on your lean mass. You will consequently potentially lose muscle and cravings while stopping to draw on your body fat. Everything you want to avoid when you fast to improve your body composition!

I'm Drinking Coffee! Is It A Severe Doctor?

First, I am not a doctor. But my point of view is that we do not live in a perfect world. So if you choose to consume stimulants, do so knowingly: it is as if you take out an (energy) loan. When you borrow from your bank, the money you borrow will have to be paid back at some point. If you combine credits on credits, you know that you will end up having big problems. The same will apply if you take stimulants on a daily and exaggerated basis.

Sweeteners Drinks: The False Good Idea

A word also on drinks containing false sugars. We have known for a few years now that despite the absence of calories, sweeteners lure the body by stimulating the production of insulin. Their consumption, therefore, indirectly promotes insulin resistance (while fasting, on the contrary, promotes its recovery). We are not even talking here about the neurotoxic effect of these substances, which is no longer to be proven. These drinks are, therefore, entirely counterproductive in the context of intermittent fasting.

Conclusion

If you suspect chronic fatigue at home and wish to experience intermittent fasting, avoid trying to cheat by using stimulants (especially on an empty stomach), this will only slow down your results by worsening your fatigue. Once weaned from caffeine and your nervous system rested, you will have equally vital energy (if not more) on an empty stomach, and above all much more stable over time!

Do you need to wake up your metabolism in the morning? Move, breathe, walk, run, and swim! Natural stimulations will produce more beneficial and lasting results over time than purely chemical and addictive stimulation of caffeine. Currently, in summer, I like the contact with cold water every morning. This puts me in good condition for the rest of the day. It's up to you to find what suits you!

Mistake Number 2: Wanting To Do Too Much

Many people go headlong into the single meal mode because they have been told that it is the best of the best that they will live ten times longer and lose a hundred times more fat. As often, the excess of enthusiasm hides a more nuanced reality.

In reality, you will only get results that match what your body can currently support, depending on your level of vitality. **There is only one rule: you must feel good.** If you are calm and concentrated at the same time, and you do not feel hunger at all, these are signs that your body is drawing in its fats. You can continue to fast (and you do it naturally because it is easy for you).

But if on the other hand, you start to be stressed for no apparent reason, to have difficulty concentrating, to be irritable, to have obsessive thoughts for food, this is undoubtedly the sign that you have exceeded your capacity for adaptation (to the lack of glucose), your cortisol levels get carried away, and your stress level can potentially become destructive. You can also recognize yourself in this description if, when you are refueling, you experience hyperplasic disorders. **The problem is not intermittent fasting, but the fact that you have set the bar too high.**

Being too rigid on schedules can be counterproductive.

I noticed how my ability to fast was reduced to nothing if, for one reason or another, I went through a period of fatigue, lack of sleep. In this case, I do not feel guilty, and I eat to get fuel and do my daily activities. Conversely, when I am well-rested, I can sometimes eat nothing until the evening without even thinking about it. Intermittent fasting is a great tool, but it is not magical and should not become a religion. You do not have to practice it strictly 365 days a year to get the benefits.

Note that I am not speaking here of therapeutic fasting in the classical sense of the term. The purposes are not precisely the same. In intermittent, daily fasting, we aim to optimize metabolism above all and wish to remain active.

And What about the Warrior Diet?

You can consume during the day a small portion of foods with a low glycemic index (example: a handful of berries, a glass of vegetable juice), meals with little digestive impact, and in small quantities. This approach is notably recommended by Ori Hofmekler, author of the **"Warrior Diet"** and one of the people known to have significantly contributed to popularizing intermittent fasting in our modern era.

If you choose to test the Warrior Diet, don't forget the keyword: **control**. The risk in adopting this strategy is to generate cravings for compulsive snacking and to cancel the benefits of the period of restriction. Indeed, even fruits and vegetable juices can cause a significant rise in blood sugar, and therefore, insulin is not a problem in absolute terms. Still, when you fast, you want to keep your insulin as low as possible to prevent burning your fat stores.

So, is the –Warrior Diet‖ for you? If you can control yourself and settle for a handful of berries without waking you up for the rest of the day, why not? Otherwise, in my experience, it is better to reserve fruits and vegetables during the feeding window and do a speedy the rest of the time.

Example of fruits with a low glycemic index.

Conclusion

If you exceed your adaptability by wanting to push the fast too far in the day, you risk obtaining the opposite effects of those sought. Go gradually to start skipping (or just selling) breakfast. For example, the body needs time to learn how to use its fat stores. Wanting to go too fast means taking the risk of spending your days without the energy to depress and ultimately give up. Play and progress with intermittent fasting without making it a dogma.

Mistake Number 3: Not Eating Enough after Breaking the Fast

As much as you must be on a food restriction during the fasting phase, as much during the compensation phase, **you must eat enough and to the full, whether in one or more doses**. Do not be afraid of eating enough in the evening, thinking that you are going to store fat. It is a legend linked to the fact that most people snack all day long. Limiting yourself in the evening in the latter context will have an impact beneficial. But when we fast a significant part of the day, we are in a completely different meaning.

Be careful, and it is, of course, not a question of gorging yourself and gobbling up everything that comes your way, especially just before sleeping, at the risk of spending your night (poorly) digesting. Eating in serenity with proper chewing is always a must. If you cannot control yourself, I refer you to the previous point.

Intermittent fasting also does not slow down the metabolism in the long term as we sometimes hear it in the mouths of its detractors. Once again, if we eat enough during the compensation phase.

Do not make restrictions during the compensation phase.

How Do I Know If I'm eating enough with one or Two Meals a Day?

If you are doing the –single meal‖ mode (4 to 6-hour food window, for example), think about large family meals or when you go to a restaurant. **Take your time!** A –single meal‖ does not necessarily mean a single plate or a single food intake. A little tip from Ori: allow at least 20 to 30 minutes (or more) to pass after each food intake, the time generally necessary for the signal of satiety to rise to the brain. If hunger returns after this time, you can continue eating. However, avoid eating all of your calories just before sleeping for reasons that you will quickly understand (digestion).

Conclusion

One of the main benefits of intermittent fasting is that it allows you to reconnect with your real hunger. Learn to listen to it without locking yourself into overly complicated protocols that don't suit your needs. The quality of your **digestion**, your **sleep**, as well as your **energy** and your **mood** daily being four good indicators allowing you to know if you are doing things the right way or not.

Chapter 3:
What to Eat While Intermittent
Fasting: Recipes

Breakfast

1. Berries and a Tablespoon of Yogurt

About the wellbeing, berries have astounding notoriety. Blueberries are stuffed with cell reinforcements, called anthocyanins, that may help keep memory sharp as you age, and raspberries contain ellagic corrosive, a compound with hostile to malignancy properties. All berries are incredible wellsprings of fiber, a supplement significant for a sound stomach related framework. Yet, if you need more motivations to delve into summer's sun-kissed little organic products, look no farther than two new examinations, which recommend that berries might be useful for your heart and your bones also. In an investigation of 72 middle-age individuals distributed as of late in the American Journal of Clinical Nutrition, eating directly under a cup of blended berries every day for about two months was related with expanded degrees of —good‖ HDL cholesterol and brought down circulatory strain, two positives with regards to heart wellbeing.

Remembered for the blend were strawberries, red raspberries, and bilberries-like blueberries-just as different berries increasingly regular in Finland (where the examination was led): dark currants, lingonberries, and choke¬berries. -Right now we don't realize which berry, or berries, could have been the most dynamic,‖ says Iris Erlund, Ph.D., senior scientist at the National Public Health Institute in Helsinki and lead creator of the investigation. Be that as it may, truth be told, the various scope of the polyphenols-an expansive class of wellbeing advancing plant exacerbates that incorporates anthocyanins, and ellagic corrosive gave by the blend of berries is likely answerable for the watched benefits. Polyphenols may expand levels of nitric oxide, a particle that creates various heart-solid impacts.

One is assisting with loosening up veins, which in this manner brings about brought down circulatory strain, says Erlund. Polyphenols may likewise help safeguard with boning thickness after menopause, as per new research in the Journal of Nutritional Biochemistry. Our bones are continually –turning over‖ - separating down and working back. After menopause, when estrogen levels plunge, bone breakdown outpaces bone development, and the outcome is a bone misfortune, a hazard factor for osteoporosis. In the investigation, rodents that had their ovaries expelled (to mirror an estrogen-denied postmenopausal state) and were bolstered blueberries consistently for a quarter of a year mainly expanded their bone thickness, researchers at Florida Study University found. –We accept that polyphenols in the berries eased back the rate [of bone turnover], eventually sparing bone,‖ says Bahram Arjmandi, Ph.D., R.D., the investigation's lead creator and teacher and seat of the division of sustenance, nourishment and exercise sciences at FSU. More research is hard to know without a doubt whether the advantages mean people at the same time, says Arjmandi, the information proposes that eating even a modest quantity of blueberries every day-maybe as meager as 1/4 cup-could be useful for anybody's bones.

Yogurt is staple nourishment in a few societies, beginning from nations in Western Asia and the Middle East. The word yogurt is accepted to be gotten from the Turkish word –yoğurmak,‖ which intends to thicken, coagulate, or turn sour. [1] Historical records portray roaming herders are conveying milk in pockets made of creature skins. Usually, happening proteins in the pockets that were transmitted near the body created enough body warmth to age the milk, delivering consumable nourishment that endured longer than milk; along these lines, the presentation of yogurt!. Extra sorts of lactobacilli and bifid bacteria might be included. The microbes convert the sugar in milk, called lactose, to lactic corrosive, which thickens the milk and builds up its particular tart flavor. References to yogurt and wellbeing go back to 6000 BCE, as found in Indian Ayurvedic restorative writings. He additionally inquired about the specific wellbeing impacts of lactic corrosive.

Today, yogurt can be found in an assortment of structures—including plain, yet frequently with included organic products or sugars. Thickeners and stabilizers, for example, gelatin and gelatins, may likewise be added for a thicker surface and more extravagant taste. People with lactose narrow mindedness who can't endure dairy items might have the option to eat some yogurt in light of its lower grouping of lactose. Maturation by the microbes separates lactose to lactic corrosive. Another alternative might be plant-based yogurts, which don't contain lactose.

2. ¼ Cup Heated Beans on Toast

Beans may get negative criticism for making individuals gassy, yet that is no motivation to remove them from your eating routine. Specialists prescribe you devour up to 3 cups of the vegetables seven days—since they are so useful for your wellbeing. What's more, the more you eat, the more outlandish you are to experience stomach difficulty. ─Individuals who eat beans on a reliable premise experience less gas and swelling than individuals who expend them less frequently,‖ says Cynthia Sass, MPH, RD, Health's contributing nourishment manager and creator of Slim down Now: Shed Pounds and Inches with Real Food, Real Fast ($20; amazon.com).

You have such a significant number of assortments to browse—dark beans, naval force beans, and kidney beans to give some examples. Peruse on to discover why they're so useful for your wellbeing, and scrumptious better approaches to make them. Fiber enables your body to feel full, so you don't have to eat as much for the day. While current dietary rules suggest ladies get around 25 grams of fiber daily, many miss the mark. By and large, ladies expend only 12.1 to 13.8 grams daily.

I hope to beans to assist you with arriving at your objective. Only a half cup of cooked naval force beans contains about 10 grams of fiber. That implies it won't wear off a lot, much after you cook them. Furthermore, seeds have the thread in both the skin and the tissue. Beans contain both solvent and insoluble fiber, so they work twofold to keep your stomach related framework running efficiently. The first hinders processing, which gives you that full inclination and the subsequent forestalls clogging. Furthermore, beans aren't as terrible for gas as you might suspect.

An examination in the Nutrition Journal took a gander at the impacts of pinto beans and dark beans on the GI tract. Members ate a half cup of either grain each day for three weeks. Even though somewhat less than half detailed expanded tooting in the first week, the vast majority of them felt it had scattered by the third week. Make sure to drink bunches of water—you need it to enable such fiber to travel through your GI tract, Sass says. Over being high in fiber, most beans additionally score low on the glycemic list, a positioning of nourishments dependent on how they influence glucose. That helps keep your glucose consistent—one explanation beans are thought to help keep diabetes under control. An examination in the Archives of Internal Medicine even found that individuals with type 2 diabetes who expended one cup of beans day by day for three weeks had the option to keep up lower glucose and pulse than when they began the eating routine. Significant levels of LDL cholesterol (the awful kind) can adhere to the dividers of your veins, causing aggravation and plaque development.

A sound cardiovascular framework begins with what you eat, and beans are one low-fat nourishment you need in your group. Considerably more motivation to get in at any rate 3/4 cup each day: an examination in the Canadian Medical Journal found that eating one serving of beans, peas, chickpeas, or lentils day by day can lessen your LDL levels by 5% and your odds of creating cardiovascular sickness by 5 to 6%. An eating routine wealthy in beans is uplifting news for your heart. At that point, there's their high fiber content. An investigation in the British Medical Journal took a gander at the connection between fiber admission and coronary illness just as a cardiovascular ailment. Specialists found that getting in an extra 7 grams of fiber for every day could fundamentally bring down your danger of growing either condition by 9%.

The magnesium then again helps in nerve capacity and circulatory strain guidelines, as indicated by the National Institutes of Health. Notwithstanding paunch filling fiber, beans are stacked with protein, another supplement that controls yearnings. While numerous individuals go to meat for their protein fix, most don't understand that beans are supplied with the supplement as well. A half-cup of cooked dark beans, for instance, contains almost 8 grams of protein. Stunningly better, the low-fat nature of beans makes it simpler for you to shed pounds. A ton of that has to do with how beans get handled in your framework — more motivation to make beans your superfood for weight reduction. Iron lack is the most widely recognized nourishing inadequacy in the United States and the primary source of whiteness, a condition where the body has a lower-than-ordinary red platelet check. Current rules propose ladies get around 18 milligrams of iron a day, yet many miss the mark regarding that objective.

Eating beans is one approach to begin on boosting your iron admission: a half cup of cooked lentils, for example, has 3.3 milligrams. In any case, since beans are plant nourishment, they contain non-home iron, which isn't as promptly ingested as the home iron you find in meat. For better retention, it's suggested you eat beans with nourishments high in nutrient C. Ttomatoes, and citrus. In many bean assortments, you'll discover thiamin, niacin, riboflavin, B6, and folate—B nutrients that assist you with changing over nourishment to vitality, support high cholesterol, and lessen irritation, in addition to other things. Research has demonstrated that folate and B6 might be useful for bringing down your danger of cardiovascular illness, as well.

A Japanese report in Stroke found that higher utilization of folate and B6 was related to fewer passings from a cardiovascular breakdown in men, in addition to fewer crossings from stroke, coronary illness, and all-out cardiovascular occasions in ladies. While you can likewise get your admission of B nutrients from fish, entire grains, and veggies, adding beans to your eating regimen is an extraordinary method to prop your body up securely. Beans are wealthy in cancer prevention agents, which ensure against free radicals that could harm your cells and lead to malignant growth.

Ladies who ate beans or lentils at any rate two times each week more than eight years were less inclined to create bosom malignant growth than the individuals who just ate them once per month or less in an investigation of more than 90,000 ladies distributed in the International Journal of Cancer. Another survey in The Journal of Cancer Research discovered ladies who expended at least four servings of vegetables seven days had a lower occurrence of colorectal polyps, an antecedent to both colon and rectal malignancies. Other characteristic substances in beans could likewise have an impact on battling the disease — only one more motivation to give more love.

3. Touch plate of mixed greens with fish

Fish is a magnificent wellspring of top-notch proteins and omega-3 unsaturated fats. It additionally adds to the admission of supplements, for example, iodine, selenium, calcium, iron, and nutrients An and D. Omega-3 unsaturated fats, DHA (docosahexaenoic corrosive) and EPA (eicosapentaenoic corrosive) are found in each sort of fish, however, are particularly high in greasy fish (for example salmon and yellow croaker) Omega-3 unsaturated fats help bring down the danger of coronary illness and stroke and are significant for fetal neurological improvement.

While calcium and nutrient D are substantial in creating healthy teeth and bones, iodine is required for the creation of thyroid hormones. An inadequacy of iodine in the eating routine is related to the improvement of goiter and captured development. Fish is additionally a wellspring of introduction to contaminants like dioxins, PCBs, and mercury. In any case, past CFS examines have affirmed that it is improbable for the nearby populace to encounter, through the utilization of nourishment, bothersome wellbeing impacts of dioxins and PCBs, including NDL-PCBs.

Furthermore, numerous abroad investigations have announced a decrease in the degree of these contaminants in fish throughout the years. Methylmercury is the natural type of mercury and can unfavorably influence the sensory system in the creating baby.

Studies have demonstrated that some native fish species may contain high methylmercury levels, which are hence a worry for ladies of kid bearing age. Also, little youngsters whose minds are as yet creating might be more defenseless than grown-ups to the unfriendly impacts of methylmercury, which remember a decrease in IQ.

Lunch

1. Grass-Bolstered Liver Burgers

Liver. You know its bravo. Customary cookbooks incorporate plans for liver pates that are loaded up with enticing portrayals like —rich,‖ —lavish,‖ and —smooth.‖ Blogs are jumbled with dilettantish pictures of seared liver and gleaming onions dispensed onto beautiful platters. The liver, once evaded and overlooked, is presently being applauded in wellbeing networks for its ground-breaking protein substance and an extraordinary mix of nutrients. In any case, regardless of anything else that smell, that taste, that surface well, put pleasantly, the liver is only not for everybody. Along these lines, for all the offal-apprehensive out there, here is a tricky burger formula that utilizes a mystery run of the dried liver to make a simple, stable, and shockingly typical tasting feast. Because you have a waiting aversion for the liver, it doesn't imply that you are a hopeless disappointment at customary cooking.

There is by all accounts a tendency in some familial wellbeing circles to despicably shroud abhorrence's for liver, just as an aversion of this whiz nourishment some way or another uncovers you as an impostor genuine foodie. There is additionally an increasingly normal inclination for individuals to be so absolutely appalled by the liver, that they dismiss the nourishment speeding by a plate of it in the supermarket or coating over articles about its medical advantages as they don't exist. In either circumstance, the liver is disregarded, and it's necessarily not reasonable. If you don't care for the organ or are anxious about difficult it, that is entirely worthy. In any case, even still, there are approaches to get liver into the eating routine and be cheerful as well! Envision that? Everything necessary is getting more innovative about fitting this superfood into your eating routine.

2. Egg or Beans

Beans pack a great deal of fiber enables your body to feel full, so you don't have to eat as much for the day. While current dietary rules suggest ladies get around 25 grams of fiber daily, many miss the mark. By and large, ladies expend only 12.1 to 13.8 grams daily. I hope to beans to assist you with arriving at your objective. Only a half cup of cooked naval force beans contains about 10 grams of fiber. That implies it won't wear off a lot, much after you cook them.

Furthermore, beans have fiber in both the skin and the tissue. Beans are useful for assimilation Beans to contain both solvent and insoluble fiber, so they work twofold to keep your stomach related framework dashing.

The first hinders processing, which gives you that full inclination and the subsequent forestalls clogging.

Furthermore, beans aren't as terrible for gas as you might suspect. An examination in the Nutrition Journal took a gander at the impacts of pinto beans and dark beans on the GI tract. Members ate a half cup of either bean each day for three weeks. Even though somewhat less than half detailed expanded tooting in the first week, the vast majority of them felt it had scattered by the third week. Make sure to drink bunches of water—you need it to enable such fiber to travel through your GI tract, Sass says.

3. Salmon and Vegetables

Eating a routine eating wealthy in leafy foods as a feature of a general sound eating regimen may decrease the chance for stroke and maybe other cardiovascular illnesses. Eating an eating regimen wealthy in foods grown from the ground as a significant aspect of a general solid eating routine may decrease the chance for type 2 diabetes. Eating a routine eating wealthy in foods grown from the ground as a component of a general solid eating regimen may ensure against specific malignancies, for example, mouth, stomach, and colon-rectum disease.

Diets wealthy in nourishments containing fiber, for example, products of the soil, may lessen the danger of coronary illness. Eating leafy foods wealthy in potassium as a component of a general sound eating routine may diminish the risk of creating kidney stones and may assist with decreasing bone misfortune. Eating nourishments, for example, vegetables that are low in calories per cup rather than some other unhealthier nourishment might be valuable in assisting with bringing down calorie consumption.

Snacks

1. Kale and Broccoli

Broccoli is known to be a generous and delicious vegetable that is wealthy in many supplements. It is said to pack the most nourishing punch of any vegetable. At the point when we consider green vegetables to remember for our eating routine, broccoli is one of the preeminent veggies to strike a chord. Originating from the cabbage family, broccoli can be classified as a consumable green plant. Here is a portion of the advantages of broccoli:

1. Disease counteraction: Broccoli shares malignant growth battling and insusceptible, boosting properties with different cruciferous vegetables, for example, cauliflower, Brussels sprouts, and cabbage. Broccoli contains properties that exhaust estrogens, which ordinarily cause disease in the body. Research shows that broccoli is very appropriate for forestalling bosom and uterus malignancy.

2. Cholesterol decrease: Like numerous entire nourishments, broccoli is stuffed with solvent fiber that coaxes cholesterol out of your body. This is because the fiber stuck broccoli helps dilemma with bile acids in the stomach related tract. This makes discharging cholesterol out of our body simple. As indicated by an examination by the Institute of Food Research, a specific assortment of broccoli can help lessen the blood LDL-cholesterol levels by 6 percent.

3. Decreasing unfavorably susceptible response and irritation: Research has demonstrated the capacity of kaempferol to reduce the effect of hypersensitivity related substances on our body. Broccoli even has large measures of omega three unsaturated fats, which are notable as calming. Alongside this, broccoli can likewise help individuals experiencing joint inflammation as broccoli contains sulforaphane, a synthetic that hinders the catalysts that can cause joint devastation and consequently lead to irritation.

4. Broccoli is profoundly focused on nutrient C, making it incredible for resistance: Other than this, broccoli additionally contains flavonoids that help reuse the nutrient C proficiently. It is likewise advanced with carotenoids lutein, zeaxanthin, beta-carotene, and other force stuffed cancer prevention agents.

5. Bone wellbeing: Broccoli contains elevated levels of both calcium and nutrient K, the two of which are significant for bone wellbeing and counteraction of osteoporosis. Alongside calcium, broccoli is likewise loaded with different supplements like magnesium, zinc, and phosphorous. In light of these properties, broccoli is incredibly reasonable for youngsters, old and lactating moms.

6. Heart wellbeing: The mitigating properties of sulforaphane, one of the is thiocyanates (ITCs) in broccoli, might have the option to forestall (or even invert) a portion of the harm to vein linings that can be brought about by irritation because of constant glucose issues. Broccoli is extraordinary for heart wellbeing as it contains filaments, unsaturated fats, and nutrients that assist directing with blooding pressure in the body. This likewise helps in diminishing awful cholesterol, consequently prompting a sound heart. Broccoli helps to shield veins from harming too.

7. Diet help: Broccoli is a decent carb and is high in fiber, which helps in processing, forestalls obstruction, keeps up low glucose, and checks indulging. Alongside this, broccoli is likewise incredible for weight reduction since it is wealthy in fiber. It is a perfect green vegetable to remember for your servings of mixed greens and finishing your five shaded vegetables ordinary. Likewise, broccoli additionally contains proteins, making it appropriate for veggie lovers that are, in any case, not ready to finish their protein prerequisite.

8. Incredible for detoxification: Since broccoli is wealthy in fiber, it can help dispose of poisons through the stomach related tract. Other than this, broccoli is likewise brimming with cell reinforcements that help in generally speaking detoxification of the body. Broccoli incorporates unique phytonutrients that help in the body's detox procedure. Broccoli additionally contains isothiocyanates, which help in the detox procedure at the hereditary level.

9. Healthy skin: Skincare incorporates sparkle, yet additionally, its insusceptibility. Since broccoli is a powerhouse of cancer prevention agents and supplements like nutrient C and minerals such as copper and zinc, broccoli helps in keeping up a healthy skin. This implies it likewise shields the skin from getting diseases as keep the natural sparkle of your skin. Broccoli is loaded with nutrient K, amino acids, and folates, making it perfect for keeping up solid skin insusceptibility.

10. Eye care: Broccoli contains beta-carotene, nutrient A, phosphorous and different nutrients such B complex, nutrient C and E. All these rich supplements are extraordinary for eye wellbeing as this assistance in ensuring the eyes against macular degeneration, waterfall and even fixes harm done by unsafe radiations we experience by being continually on our telephones or being before a screen. 11. Hostile to maturing: Since broccoli is enhanced with nutrient C, which has various cell reinforcement properties, it is incredible for against maturing. This is because cell reinforcements help battle the free radicals liable for maturing. These free radicals regularly harm the skin. Eating broccoli routinely helps in decreasing almost negligible differences, wrinkles, skin issues like skin inflammation, and even pigmentation.

2. Nuts and Seeds

Seeds are a significant expansion to any sound eating routine – they aren't as a rule as respected as nuts, even though they unquestionably have the right to be. Loaded up with a useful commendation of essential fats, protein, an immense range of various supplements and phytonutrients, they assume a significant job in supporting wellbeing. Seeds are the epitome of general life power; each seed, a little force place of enormous potential, intended to develop into a high, bounteous plant. They are just overflowing with goodness. Seeds are a great option in contrast to nuts, frequently less rich (which I for one like), and more straightforward to process. You can discover crude shelled seeds or seed-spreads in any better than average wellbeing store. Sprouting seeds will, in general, make the supplements all the more promptly accessible for assimilation.

Growing has the extra advantage of discharging the compound inhibitors inside seeds, making them all the simpler to process. On the off chance that you have my formula book, at that point, look at the crude grew sunflower seed pesto formula – it's so energetic – one of my outright most loved plans. The released life power from becoming makes such a dynamic and staggeringly delectable dish. Seeds make superb oils, frequently somewhat lighter than nut oil. While I feel it is in every case best to appreciate an entire seed (one that despite everything has every last bit of its parts – regardless of whether ground down), oils, despite everything, offer an extraordinary method to get a portion of essential fats in your eating routine.

Hemp seed oil, and sunflower seed oil, are exceptional models that you may use as a feature of a serving of mixed greens dressing. Continuously pick the most excellent, cold, squeezed oil that you can discover. Hemp oil is my top pick. It ought to taste great (it won't feel great on the off chance that you don't purchase a decent one) and ought to have a green tint to it. Appreciate oil with some restraint – a sprinkle to a great extent, yet don't overdo it.

3. Clean Meat Sources, Vegetables, and A Few Fruits

While the present pattern is tied in with going veggie-lover, eating meat (because of the awfulness anecdotes about red meat) is quickly lessening. A great many people consider vegetables and natural products to get the job done when it comes there every day dietary needs while likewise feeling that plant protein is better (and more secure) than creature protein. As this isn't valid, here is a rundown of the medical advantages of eating meat that all add to completing indispensable metabolic capacities yet additionally giving one a ton of vitality too:

Advantage 1

Since meat contains a lot of protein, this could be valuable to the body as the requirement for protein is a significant one for the body. Since protein is said to improve the general wellbeing and prosperity of one's body, there are different advantages, for example, the fix and working of body tissues just as the creation of antibodies that will shield the body from diseases, subsequently fortifying the insusceptible framework too. Above all, since meat contains all the essential amino acids, it certainly positions as probably the best wellspring of protein.

Advantage 2

The numerous supplements that meat provides, it is wealthy in iron, zinc, and selenium. While iron aides in framing hemoglobin that transports oxygen to various pieces of your body, zinc helps in tissue arrangement and digestion, just as selenium separates the fat and synthetic compounds in the body.

Advantage 3

Nutrients are additionally a significant piece of the one's eating regimen, and Vitamin A, B, and D are usually found in meat also. Not exclusively do these nutrients advance great vision, more grounded teeth, and bones; however, it likewise bolsters the focal sensory system in this manner, improving psychological well-being also. Another significant advantage of eating meat is the support of your skin's wellbeing.

Chapter 4:
What Is Autophagy?

With the process of autophagy, our body cells build their unusable components, such as B. misfolded proteins and damaged cell components. Our cells use them to generate new building blocks or use them as fuel, similar to the energy generation from fat reserves in the event of a calorie deficit.

Emergency Program and Cell Cleaning

Autophagy is, therefore, on the one hand, an emergency system in periods of hunger and, at the same time, an essential process for cleaning and renewing the cells. This process is also what you mean when you speak colloquially of —detoxification.‖ Functioning autophagy protects against diseases such as cancer, dementia, heart disease, and bacterial infections. Degenerate cells, deposits, and malignant bacteria have a reduced chance of accumulating because they are broken down at the initial stage.

Autophagy Experiment with Mice

Researchers examined two groups of mice that were kept under the same conditions and were given the same amount of food. There was only one difference: Group 1 was fed continuously at regular short intervals. Group 2 received the same amount of food within a few hours and then had to fast the rest of the day.

The result: Group 1 consistently had thick, sluggish mice that died prematurely from a fatty liver. Group 2 consisted of lean, vital mice that had a long lifespan. Experiments of this kind were repeated many times with different organisms and always came to the same result. What happens there? It has been found that fasting or interval fasting leads to a process of cellular self-cleaning, autophagy.

Such experiments clearly show that longer intervals between meals have a considerable advantage on the vitality and lifespan of the organism. The positive effects of interval fasting are also evident for the human body. The explanation is as follows: eating too often inhibits the cell's self-cleaning process. The cell literally —garbage‖ when autophagy is prevented by constant energy replenishment from outside.

Autophagy Inhibited by Insulin

The constant increase in insulin levels from eating too often seems to inhibit cell cleaning. Insulin promotes the storage of nutrients in the body's energy reserves. If insulin is released continuously, the body receives the signal that sufficient energy is being supplied from outside and that no self-digestion is necessary. The energy reserves are not tapped but are retained. Pollutants accumulate, which is colloquially often referred to as —slagging‖ and at the same time, there is a very high risk of being overweight.

What Does Autophagy Promote in Our Cells?

- **Fasting (from approx. 14 to 17 hours; regular therapeutic fasting cures are optimal.**
- **Calorie restriction (chronic mild calorie deficit with a balanced diet)**
- **Sports (both strength and endurance sports)**

Some foods and substances: Graz researchers have succeeded in identifying foods and substances that activate cellular waste disposal even though the organism eats. This includes coffee and foods with high spermidine content (see below).

How Bose Coffee Affect Autophagy?

For example, coffee is an autophagy trigger, the scientists confirm. The tasty pick-me-up is a trendy drink in Germany with a per capita consumption of around 5.5 kg per year. Studies show that coffee has hugely positive effects on various metabolic diseases, such as diabetes or disorders of fat metabolism.

Within one to four hours after drinking coffee, autophagy in all examined organs is strongly stimulated. This also applies to decaffeinated coffee, which means that it is not due to caffeine. Still, one suspects that secondary plant substances, so-called polyphenols in coffee, have this effect. But be careful: animal protein, in turn, inhibits autophagy, so do not add cow's milk to the coffee! Only black or with a vegetable alternative such as B. Enjoyed almond milk.

Where Does the Term Autophagy Come From?

The concept of autophagy was coined in 1963 by Christian de Duve, who discovered this self-digestion process of the cell for the first time. The Japanese scientist Yoshinori Sumy was awarded the Nobel Prize in Medicine in 2016 because his research enabled him to explain the mechanisms of autophagy in more detail.

What Controls Autophagy?

Cells don't just eat themselves. This process only takes place under particular conditions and depends on complex molecular conditions. Enzymes such as mTOR and AMPK are involved, which closely monitor how many nutrients and how much energy is available to the cell. If too little of it is possible, they initiate the process of autophagy to break down old cell components that are currently not needed. The resulting parts can then be used by the body to build new and urgently needed cell components.

What Are the Tasks of Autophagy?

1. Autophagy as a Survival Mechanism

Digesting superfluous things and gaining building materials or energy from them → Autophagy thus serves as a survival mechanism in reduced times. —If cells are exposed to a lack of food, they digest everything that is not needed, and Cells can convert these —cellular garbage‖ in the energy they provide. Subsequently, the body once again available. –

2. Autophagy as Part of the Immune System and Defense Mechanism

If foreign proteins or unwanted viruses and bacteria enter the cells, they are eaten framework of autophagy and thus rendered harmless.

3. Autophagy as a Cleaning Repair Mechanism

With the many metabolic processes in our body, cell components are damaged, and defective proteins are formed. So that they do not cause problems, they are decomposed by autophagy and removed, which can lead to cell death, called apoptosis, also in the final stages.

When this cleaning process is disrupted, more and more substances are deposited in our cells, which is considered to be one of the main reasons for cell aging. One could also say that together with apoptosis, autophagy is the cellular quality control and, therefore, essential for maintaining the functionality of our cells.

Animal experiments have shown that reducing calories increases life expectancy. The reason could be the increased autophagy that causes the cell components to be broken down and rebuilt more often so that less —ballastǁ is deposited.

How Can You Activate Autophagy?

With the process of autophagy, our body cells break down their unusable components. Misfolded proteins and damaged cell components are used to generate new building blocks. Without autophagy, the cellular waste would accumulate in the cell and sooner or later would hinder the smooth functioning of the cell.

Autophagy is an essential process for cell cleansing and renewal. These prevent diseases such as cancer, dementia, heart diseases, and diabetes. Functioning autophagy is, therefore, important protection and building block for a healthy life.

We now know that there are several ways to activate autophagy. The two best-studied are interval fasting and spermidine administration.

Interval Fasting

Fasting can prolong life, rejuvenate, and regenerate by triggering autophagy. Already 16 hours of abstinence trigger this effect. This is known as interval fasting or autophagy fasting. If there is no external energy supply, cells begin to digest the harmful cell components. Dead, malformed, broken, or infected cells are also destroyed, and unusable parts are broken down. In this way, intruders such as viruses, bacteria, or other microorganisms can also be combated in the cell.

An immediate consequence of autophagy fasting is –detoxificationǀ and, in addition to more beautiful skin, a better, more vital general condition. Long-term effects include reducing the risk of developing cancer, dementia, cardiovascular diseases, or diabetes.

Discover this new gentle form of fasting for yourself and experience the different benefits of autophagy fasting and meal breaks - all-round renewal in the Peering fasting monastery.

Spermidine

Spermidine is a substance with the discovery of which Graz researchers triggered a wave of anti-aging studies worldwide. In almost all living organisms, spermidine is a component of life and plays a vital role in cell growth. In the human body, spermidine is found primarily in the male seminal fluid, where it has a life-extending effect on the sperm cells. The concentration of the body's spermidine decreases with age; for example, the decrease in human skin begins at around 30 years.

Furthermore, spermidine also occurs in many foods, such as. B. in wheat germ, fresh green pepper, mushrooms, and soybeans (especially fermented), citrus fruits (especially grapefruit).

When cells are supplied with spermidine from the outside, they behave like fasting: they stimulate autophagy strong. Aging cells and organisms are rejuvenated and live longer. Research shows that yeast cells cultured in a spermidine-rich medium lived four times, and human immune cells three times longer. Fruit flies and worms that were given a spermidine-rich diet had a 30 percent longer lifespan. Mice fed spermidine-enriched drinking water also lived significantly longer and showed fewer signs of aging. The advantage of this small molecule is that it is very stable, you can take it orally, it arrives unchanged in all organs and is not broken down by stomach acid. Due to its life-prolonging effect, spermidine is a big topic in anti-aging research and also very important in the development of medicines for serious diseases.

A spermidine-rich diet can theoretically cover the need for spermidine, but it must be carried out very consistently and continuously. Spermidine capsules or tablets are a good alternative. Since early 2019, the manufacturer TLL the Longevity Labs GmbH has been offering SPERMIDINE LIFE, the world's first natural nutritional supplement made from wheat germ extract with a high spermidine content.

How Does Autophagy Work?

With the process of autophagy, our body cells break down their unusable components. Misfolded proteins and damaged cell components are used to generate new building blocks. Without autophagy, the cellular waste would accumulate in the cell and sooner or later would hinder the smooth functioning of the cell.

Autophagy is an essential process for cell cleansing and renewal. These prevent diseases such as cancer, dementia, heart diseases, and diabetes. Functioning autophagy is, therefore, important protection and building block for a healthy life.

What Activates Autophagy?

Up to this point, you have probably already identified some activators. Here are the four most important ones:

Fasting: From 12 hours of abstinence onwards, autophagy is activated and continues to increase linearly until it reaches its absolute peak after about 2-3 days.

Calorie restriction: The Japanese are known to eat so much until they are 80% full. Autophagy plays an essential role in everyday life. If you want to lose weight or generally do not eat to the point of complete saturation, you are already taking a significant and unconscious step towards auto phagocytosis.

Sport: No matter whether aerobic sport (endurance sport) or anaerobic sport (high-intensity ball sport, CrossFit, strength training); Sport activates autophagy. One reason why the competition is recommended several times a week and keeps the body young and fit.

Certain foods and nutritional ingredients: some will be available shortly.

Activators for autophagy: activating cellular garbage disposal in everyday life

In scientific studies and practice, it is becoming increasingly clear that health benefits greatly if auto phagocytosis is given more space in everyday life.

This can be such that you have regular periods of fasting (one or more days of fasting). Intermittent fasting is a popular way to take advantage of autophagy almost every day:

Since this process is activated from around 12-16 hours, when the human growth hormone (HGH) is most strongly formed, many people like to do without breakfast and eating until lunch. There are enough hours between dinner and lunch to benefit from auto phagocytosis at night and in the morning.

However, you can also benefit from increased auto phagocytosis in addition to fasting through certain foods, nutritional ingredients, and medications:

- **Coffee 6**
- **Ketogenic diet 2**
- **Ginger 3**

- **Green tea 10**

- **Rishi (Far Eastern Medicinal Mushroom) 15**

- **Broccoli (Sulphoraphane 4)**

- **Vitamin D 8 (essential for proper and effective autophagy; approx. 80% of all Germans have a vitamin D deficiency)**

- **Turmeric and Turmeric Extract (Curcumin)**

- **Resveratrol 5 (red grapes and red wine)**

- **Melatonin (the sleep hormone; healthy sleep is essential)**

- **Spermidine (dietary supplement)**

- **Metformin and rapamycin (diabetes medication)**

Benefits of Autophagy

The actual definition of it is it's the consumption of the body's tissue as a metabolic process occurring during starvation or certain diseases. There's another definition of its destruction of damaged or redundant cellular components occurring in the vacuoles within the cell. Now when you look at these definitions, they sound a little grim. They say a little daunting we see words like starvation. We see words like a disease. We're thinking do we want to use this, and the truth is that there are so many different benefits of autophagy. We're going to get to those in just a moment. First, I want to give a brief overview, and I'm saying when we have to induce otology. I'm going to teach you that in just a moment, but we want to make sure that we're producing on top of to get the benefits when we induce it here's mostly what's happening.

There's the atopic ozone that's going to go around, and it's going to collect these broken-down cellular components.

Regulate Mitochondria Function

Now due to a lot of oxidative stress that people are coming across daily of the mitochondria, in any case, it doesn't function too well, and that's why so many people have chronic fatigue. Just a general overall lack of energy inducing artificial even up those mitochondria and help them run more efficiently, giving you more power.

Protect the Nervous System Against Injury and Disease.

It is essential for people who have Alzheimer's and their families to mention their family neurological conditions in their family so important. Improve cognitive function, and it's going to help encourage the growth of new brain cells who don't want that once again like I said if you're someone who has different neurological diseases in your family, you want to make sure you're encouraging those brain cells to grow. We also want to make sure that if we're just someone who wants to be able to have more focus and clarity that we're using ways to induce autophagy as well.

Anti-Aging and Longevity

It's going to support the growth of heart cells in the studies suggest that's going to help protect against heart disease. This is so important because heart disease is one of those top killers of people today is also going to help boost an immune.

Boost and Balance the Immune System

This is also important if we look at how many people who have hyper immunity people who are going around allergy-ridden skin rashes. All this stuff their immune systems are shot their gut is shot using fasting to help balance the immune system and improve immunity. It's going to be so powerful next thing.

Remove Pathogens and Toxins from the Cell

We live in a very, very toxic world today that bio and all these toxins bio accumulate in the body using these methods can help clear them out.

Protect DNA

It also is going to help protect the DNA and then lastly and probably most importantly for a lot of us is going to help fight against disease if you're someone who has cancer in your family. If someone who has neurological disorders in your family fasting and otology is an absolute must, it is so important. The research shows again that this natural method will help reduce the risk of these diseases, and you know if you've seen your family go through this, you certainly don't want to I know that I've seen many of my family members go through cancer go through dementia. It's horrible to not only have to live through, but it's also horrific to watch, so we'll make sure that we're using these methods.

Fasting

First on our list is going to be fasting, and many of you know about this, so when we look at the research of how fast and can induce a tiff to achieve. Basically what the research is showing us is that for the best results it's going to start at about 24 hours, so you're going to have to fast for about 24 hours and then move forward from there and so if we want the best results with autophagy to think of 24 hours plus. A lot of people go and do three days fast for a fast seven day fast. That's where you're going to get the absolute most benefit I'm going to move on, but I'll circle back to fasting in telling you how you can get better results in shorter fasting hours.

Get Kato-Adapted

Some studies suggest ketosis can cause starvation-induced otology. A lot of people are following the ketogenic diet today for a lot of good reasons. It's helping them improve their quality of life and improve their health overall now if we use the ketogenic diet.

Exercise

Exercise basically what they found is that those who exercise have higher otology related markers of gene activities. So what this is saying is this you're someone who is applied regularly let's say five days a week for five-ten plus years mainly. You're going to have higher amounts of staff-related markers of gene activity and so exercising. We know it is good, but if you're using on the regular, it's even better we're also going to look at exercise as a way to help induce otology in another way.

One study suggests that exercise-induced auto fatigue in multiple organs muscles the liver pancreas and adipose tissue, and so when we take these different methods, and we combine them. We're going to get the best results, and that's why we're I'm going to circle back to fasting, so if we are fasting and we're doing the ketogenic diet, and we're exercising. You're going to be able to induce ontology in a much shorter period some research suggests that some people can do it in 14 16 hours. So utilizing multiple methods to induce autophagy stacking those natural methods, you're going to get better results even from there, so we want to make sure that not only do we utilize fasting but some of these other methods to help them.

What Triggers Autophagy?

Fasting Triggers Autophagy

The cellular —Geisel evacuation‖ is mainly stimulated by controlled fasting. But according to the latest findings, diets have also been identified that turn on the molecular effects of fasting even though you eat. This means that it is not necessary to fast for several days to get autophagy going.

Intermittent fasting (overnight fasting, for example, with an early dinner and a late breakfast) is enough to stimulate autophagy. Autophagy is intensified by drinking coffee in the morning (NOT in the evening). It has been scientifically confirmed that within one to four hours after consuming coffee in the model organisms, the cellular autophagy of all the organs examined - liver, skeletal muscles, and heart - was significantly boosted. By the way, the effect is independent of whether the coffee is caffeine or decaffeinated, because the stimulation of autophagy does not seem to be the caffeine itself. The result probably comes from secondary plant substances (polyphenols).

Coffee without Milk and Sugar

Animal proteins (e.g., cow's milk) in coffee inhibit cell cleaning (autophagy). However, herbal alternatives like almond milk do not affect autophagy. Therefore: Enjoy coffee with a clear conscience, but preferably black or with vegetable-based dairies, such as almond or coconut milk.

Attention: During the fasting phase, however, any carbohydrates should be avoided to stay in fat metabolism.

Coffee also has very positive effects on various metabolic diseases, such as diabetes, disorders of fat metabolism, etc. But coffee is not coffee - good coffee tastes good without milk and sugar. Choose the best organically grown gently roasted coffee!

Which Triggers or Foods Can Activate Autophagy?

In principle, autophagy is permanently active and is concerned with breaking down and recycling the molecular waste in our cells. However, it can be strengthened by certain stimuli in the body. This includes, for example, fasting. But we can also stimulate autophagy sustainably or, unfortunately, disrupt it through our diet. Many researchers in Germany are currently working on this finding. For example, some foods support autophagy as well as foods that can interfere with the process of autophagy.

In this context, foods with molecule spermidine are particularly attractive. The anti-aging effect of this active ingredient was discovered in 2009 by a research group led by Dr. Frank Madeo (University of Graz) recognized, see: Fuel for the brain.

A lot of spermidine is found in wheat germ, wheat bran, grapefruit, and soybeans. Other foods with reasonably high spermidine content are:

- **Broccoli**
- **Green beans**
- **Mushrooms**
- **Mangos**
- **Fermented cheese such as Cheddar**

You can find a detailed article about a wheat germ on my website gesundheit-speisen.de.

Auch coffee can happily enhance autophagy. Unfortunately, this only works if you drink coffee without milk.

Animal protein, unfortunately, inhibits the process of autophagy. Plant milk may be an alternative to cow's milk.

Intermittent Fasting and Autophagy

It is not possible to calculate precisely when autophagy starts from a fasting period. Many individual factors play a role here. In some people, autophagy may start after a short fast of 8 hours. In other people, it may take 10 to 12 hours. In any case, it has now been scientifically proven that regular fasting has a positive effect on autophagy. The interval fasting is indeed in my fasting forum more interesting - not least because of several books that have been published in recent years on this subject:

- **Eating breaks: Better than any diet!**
- **Healthy and slim thanks to short-term fasting**

- **Intermittent fasting**

- **The Fast Diet - The Original: Eat five days, fast for two days**

- **The "Tomorrow I can eat what I want" diet**

- **The 5: 2 diet: eat five days - 2 days diet**

- **The 1-day diet**

Die autophagy may, for example, more quickly started when the sport is at play because a sporting activity also leads to a nutrient deficiency occurs in our body cells.

Chapter 5:
Intermittent Fasting for Anti-Aging

As the popularity of fasting is increasing over time, further research has revealed that the benefits of eating and drinking can be much higher than just losing weight. Some research is showing to us that intermittent fasting can play an essential role in changing the symptoms of aging and aging. Let's research some recent research on how intermittent fasting can help lead a longer and healthier life.

What Is Intermittent Fasting?

Fasting is one of the popular health trends in the world. People are using intermittent fasting to lose weight and regain control of their health. This includes a meal time restriction that provides for eating and fasting periods. Fasting is not a traditional diet, as it is not changing what you are eating, but it is a pattern of food that you write at your meal.

A regular fasting schedule is to include all your meals between 12-8 hours in the evening, which means you fast for 16 hours and eat 8 hours a day. This is known as 16/8.

Intermittent fasting is known to be an effective weight-loss intervention. But did you know that further research reveals that intermittent fasting can also help with many other markers of health, including aging? These are three ways that intermittent fasting can help you to live longer.

Anti-Aging Benefits of Intermittent Fasting

There are three main benefits of intermittent fasting, which we discuss below.

- **Intermittent Fasting Increases Ketones**
- **Hormesis**
- **Fasting Triggers Autophagy**

Intermittent Fasting Increases Ketones

In the fasting state, the body is deprived of glucose, which is usually consumed by carbohydrates and proteins. The body's preferred source of energy is glucose, but when fasting, the body is forced to use alternative sources of fuel. In the absence of glucose, the body breaks down the fat in the liver and converts the grease into an available source of energy called ketones.

Ketones are locked in the mitochondria and used as fuel for the brain, heart, and muscles. Some parts of the body (especially the mind) cannot use ketones and do not require glucose. This is supplied by a process called glycogenesis, along with glucose protein deficiency. There are some benefits to aging, and we can use Alzheimer's disease as a good example. Alzheimer's disease is related to glucose metabolism.

This is why Alzheimer's disease is called type 3 diabetes. Ketones provide direct energy to the brain, avoiding deficiencies over glucose metabolism. Or improve the cognitive function of people with Alzheimer's disease, a study has reported that people with mild cognitive impairment (MCI) have increased memory of ketosis, often called Alzheimer's disease.

In this study, 23 older adults with MCI were assigned either a high carb or ketogenic diet. After six weeks, high ketone levels showed a positive correlation with memory. Other emerging evidence suggests that Alzheimer's disease in ketone beta-hydroxybutyrate (BHB) animal models Protect against Yi. Dietary changes can improve memory in older people with impaired cognitive impairment. Thus, it would make sense that intermittent fasting, which stimulates ketosis, may also help reduce mental aging.

Hormesis

Evidence suggests that regular intermittent fasting causes cells to undergo cellular stress [R]. It helps to be more flexible. This is due to the cellular flexibility hormones, a process that describes the biological response to stress. Two examples of Hermes are exercise and the use of vegetables. Activity in plants and some phytochemicals can cause a degree of importance to the body.

However, exercise and vegetables are beneficial, as the response to this stress is positive. Fasting is also an example of horseshoes. Fasting too much will cause catabolization of your muscle tissue and, eventually, death. However, a bit of stress daily to avoid the adverse effects of stress and over time can lead to positive biological reactions that increase your resilience to oxidative stress, which is one of the essential factors that affect aging. And contributes to the underlying disease.

Fasting Triggers Autophagy

Autophagy comes from a Greek word meaning food itself. Autophagy is the self-recycling of cellular waste, a process that enhances stress response. As we age, autophagy slows down, and our ability to recycle cells under stress has diminished. By fasting, we can increase autophagy, which can reduce the rate of aging because we are determined to help our body cope with cellular stress.

One study showed that relatively short-term fasting (24-48 hours) stimulated deep neurological autophagy. But the question is: Does the regular interval fasting length (16-23 hours) also affect autophagy? To date, research on fasting and autophagy has focused on 24-48 hours of fasting. This is based on the argument that autophagy usually increases in parallel to ketosis, which takes 24-48 hours to induce.

However, ketosis can be much quicker than 24 hours, and even a ketogenic diet is seen without fasting, making it theoretically possible that intermittent fasting may increase ketosis, and As a result, autophagy.

Chapter 6:
How to Lose Weight after 50 Years Old

I'll be share with you my six rules for losing weight is a multi-billion dollar industry, and there is a tendency to make things way more complicated than they need to be I think it's because people are always looking for that magic formula that's going to let them lose weight once and for all. But you don't need a magic formula. You don't need to fancy panty new-fangled ways to diet.

It's just six painless and straightforward rules that you can follow along with any eating program really, and it will optimize your weightless results, so let's get straight into it reads.

Rule Number One

That's eating as much as you can over low energy density foods low energy density means a small number of calories for a high volume of food. So the foods you should focus on eating as much of as possible ah no starchy vegetables broccoli asparagus start leafy greens like spinach rocket and kale low sugar fruits all berries are fantastic and citrus fruits broth-based soups of herbs and spices and a perfect one is air-popped popcorn your absolute best strategy for weight loss is to eat as much of all these foods as possible. You'll be packing your meals with antioxidants vitamins minerals and fiber.

Rule Number Two

You have to eat what you love okay there's no point trying to stick to a diet say paleo if you don't like meat or low-carb if your favorite foods are rice, pasta, and bread. If you're not eating foods that you really enjoy and look forward to eating, there's no way you're going to be able to stick to this diet. So it's not going to work for you no matter how good a diet it's.

Rule Number Three

You need to practice portion control; it doesn't matter how nutritious and tasty for you. Our food is if you overeat of anything, you might find it hard to lose weight. The problem is there's a vast difference between what most people consider to be a typical serving and what the right serving size is. So, it might be helpful when you're starting to lose weight get out your little kitchen scales I mean measuring cups and measure out an actual standard serving of each food.

Then you'll be able to eyeball what an excellent service look on the packet, and if they say a serve — for example, this one cup measure out that Cup.

Rule Number Four

Drink lots of herbal tea. I recommend herbal teas because one they have no calories; you have them without milk or sugar. Because they're hot, they take a long time to drink, so they fill you up.

They're a lot more satisfying than just drinking water and three they taste good they come in so many different flavors when you drink herbal tea after a meal it's going to make you feel a lot more satisfied eating this food.

Rule Number Five

My personal favorite if you're going to splurge, make sure you only splurge when you're eating out. If you splurge at home, you know it's far too easy to eat the entire contents of your kitchen. But if you go out to eat in a restaurant or at someone's house. There are natural limits imposed on you because you can only eat what you're served, and you'll pay for it. I choose so you're not going to be able to eat as much as if you were eating at home.

So, if you go out to a restaurant or go out to someone's house, make it a free meal, eat whatever you feel like eating, eat your favorite foods, enjoy yourself, and as long as you only splurge one time per week, you will lose weight.

Rule Number Six

Move your body now. Food is, by far, the essential factor in the weight-loss equation. You can lose weight without doing any exercise at all but for maximum success and to lose weight as quickly and painlessly as possible. I do suggest you get more active. This doesn't mean that you have to go crazy and do some insane amount of working out every day. It just means do more activity than you're currently doing.

So those are my six rules for losing weight.

Intermittent Fasting
16/8

A Quick Start Guide For Every Age And Stage To Fight Bad Nutrition, Reduce Belly Fat, Overcome Hunger Attacks, And Discover How To Lose Weight Without Dieting.

Introduction

How Do You Do Intermittent Fasting?

I'm going to be talking with you about fasting and, more particularly, intermittent fasting. Now intermittent fasting is something I do. It has many different benefits, including:

- Weight loss.
- Detoxification.
- Reducing bloating.
- Improving digestion.
- And much more.

So, you've probably heard of plain old traditional fasting. I mean, it's mentioned in many things throughout history, including a lot of religious books. So, you can do that kind of fasting where you only consume water for one to three days, or you can do it where you only have one meal a day again for one to three days. You can do a juice cleanse or juice fast where you only drink fruit and vegetable juice still for one to three days. With those kinds of fasting after about three days, it becomes pretty hard on your body, and so at that point, it's no longer beneficial to your health.

Now intermittent fasting gives you all the benefits of fasting while allowing you to get enough nutrition for your system. So that's why you're able to keep it up for one to three months rather than date. Here's how it works, so we're going to fast or not consume anything except water for a certain period every day. Now don't go crazy with this. We still want a pretty decent window for eating around four to eight hours, during which time we can fit a few meals.

Personally, my eating window is between seven and eight hours. So, I'll have my first meal of breakfast at around twelve. Then three I might have lunch snack at five and dinner between seven and eight. I have a longer eating window because this is a lifestyle for me. You know it's not a temporary diet that I can only sustain for one to three months; this is long-term.

But of course, if you want to have faster results, you can shorten, you're eating window to around four hours and do that for one to three months. What this shorter eating schedule does is it allows our gut to rest a lot of us will get up at safe 7:00 in the morning, eat our first meal immediately and then continue feeding throughout the day until maybe even 10:00 p.m.

If we continue to snack after dinner, so our digestive systems never have any time to rest, it's like when you finish working out, and you're supposed to let your muscles relax and heal. But we never give that to our guts. It's like we only give it maybe eight hours a day. But when we only eat for four to eight hours a day, we're giving our gut a 16 to 20-hour rest, which improves digestion, which can reduce bloating, which will give you a flatter tummy. Now one of the best benefits of intermittent fasting is that it can balance your hormone, and it can increase your body's production of human growth hormone by 400%. Now human growth hormone isn't just for growing kids and teens; it's the primary fat-burning hormone, and it helps:

- Prevent muscle loss.
- Increases muscle strength.
- Anti-aging.
- Improve your mood.
- Cognitive function.

Another way to increase HGH, which is what week school kids are calling human growth hormone, is by doing hit workout. We've talked about when to eat, but what about what to eat when doing intermittent fasting. You're going to want to make sure you get a lot of: -

- Healthy protein.
- Fat fiber.
- Eat a lot of nutrient-dense fruit.
- Eat a lot of nutrient-dense vegetables.

So pretty much you're going to want to do the ketogenic or keto diet.

How Much Weight Can You Lose Doing Intermittent Fasting?

How much weight can you lose doing intermittent fasting? In the last five months, I've lost 70 pounds doing intermittent fasting, but the answer to the question depends on the model that you're using. I'm sure it depends on your metabolism. Of course, what you're eating so.

I'll tell you a little bit about what's worked for me and what my expectations are for myself because I've come to learn that my weight loss is very formulaic and is dependent on well what I'm eating and when I'm eating. So, I eat in a one-hour window a day, and I eat one meal in that one hour so for 23 hours I'm not eating and for one hour I am eating.

I'm eating a meal that is very low in carbohydrates; it tends to be loaded with vegetables and includes some protein. In my experience, this approach has been by far the best weight loss method I've been on save like a water fast, which jump-started my whole five-month experience. I was on 16-day water quickly in the very beginning, but aside from that, this eating in a one-hour window has been beneficial.

In my case, I can lose 10 to 15 pounds a month doing this fast, and that range is dependent on what I'm eating each day. For comparison, I lost 20 pounds in the four months before this program, and it was all low-carb, and I was losing at the rate of 4 to 5 pounds a month. So, about a pound a week and so that's just from a regular low-carb diet. I was eating very similar things, but it wasn't within that one-hour window. Now I'm losing more than twice that amount, and so my weight loss is far more rapid with the one-hour eating window.

My range is from about 10 pounds to 15 pounds a month. What I find is that I can lose closer to 15 pounds a month if my one meal a day is relatively calorie-restricted. If my meal a day is more in the 500-calorie range, then I'm going to lose closer to 15 pounds in that month. If it's more in the thousand calorie range, I'm going to drop closer to 10 pounds a month.

I mean to me that's every I don't know ten days, or so it's not a lot of meals. But at home, sometimes, if I want to incorporate something you see a lot of extra fat salmon cheese's the meals are closer to a thousand calories. I have some delicious filling meals that are 500 calories, and I'm going to post some of those 500 calorie recipes for you to give you some ideas in case you haven't thought of some of these things because you know 15 pounds a month. I mean, that's a stinking a lot of weight right. I can't even believe it; I've never lost that much weight on any diet.

Of course, the water fasting and so obviously if you need to lose weight faster may be for health reasons or some other consideration. I can quickly lose the 15 pounds if I'm doing that so as you know. You eat a thousand calories every other day, and you eat zero every other day. It's not very difficult to do a 48-hour fast right now I'm not doing it. Because I feel like a little need a little bit more daily nutrition and so, I'm going back and forth between lower-calorie meals and then the thousand calorie meals.

I'm just making sure I'm always taking a liquid vitamin and mineral supplement.

Why Does Intermittent Fasting Work?

Intermittent fasting is a simple concept that is practically defined by its name; it involves incorporating periods of fasting into your diet now. The length of time for intermittent fasting varies. But a popular time frame is 16-8, meaning that you fast for 16 hours and consume all of your calories within an eight-hour eating window. This method of timing you're eating has proven to be very useful for even stubborn metabolisms. But to appreciate why it works, we need to take a fresh look at how weight loss happens. We used to think that the calorie in calorie out model was how we lost weight.

This meant that all calories were equal, so a hundred calories of meat same 200 calories of cake, which equals 200 calories of salad. When you consumed those calories, they went into a collective bucket in your body and sat there until you needed some energy at which time the calories in the bucket were released and burned the logic was that you burn more calories. Then you consume, and weight loss happened in that model of how the body burned fat seemed logical.

It didn't seem to work. The calories in the calories out model have been the predominant way of thinking for the past 60 years, which was a period that was marked by skyrocketing obesity rates. The reason it doesn't work. Because calories are not simply dumped into a collective bucket in our bodies. Instead, they are directed into two separate storage containers and store it as either glycogen or fat. The movement into those storage containers is controlled by a hormone called insulin.

So, insulin shows up when food is coming in, and when insulin is present, food energy is being stored not released. Which is vital food energy moves in one direction at a time? It's either being saved or being released. It all depends on how much insulin is present is an easy-to-access container because it is permanently stored glucose, which is very easy for your body to burn.

But this glycogen container is small. You only have about 2,000 calories of available energy stored as glycogen fat. On the other hand, it has a lot of energy; just one pound of fat has about

3500 calories worth of energy. But that is hard to access for your body to go to the trouble of burning body fat for energy. Two things must happen; you must be running low on glycogen and have a low level of insulin in your blood.

How do you get to that state you stretch out the time between meals? In other words, you follow an intermittent fasting strategy if you are frequently eating throughout the day? You are continually refilling glycogen stores and bumping up insulin. Because there is a constant supply of glycogen, there's no need for your body to go to the trouble of converting fat into energy even if your body wanted to burn fat. It can't access it because the insulin level never drops to a point where fat can be released. When you stretch out the time between meals by practicing intermittent fasting, your body burns through some of the storage of glycogen and insulin levels drop, making that a logical choice for your body to run on now.

What Can I Eat During Intermittent Fasting?

When I do get hungry usually around the 16-hour mark after yesterday's meal or around 1:00 p.m. With this example, I've got a couple of options for what we'll call lunch even though technically it's breakfast. So, if I did not have a rocket fuel latte or a bone broth to extend the fast, I'll usually have one with this lunch bacon asparagus cooked in bacon grease kimchi and a rock a few lattes. It's relatively light, but we'll also make and keep you full for a pretty long time.

If I did have a rocket fuel latte or bone broth to extend my fast in the morning, I'd usually want more volume when breaking my fast with something like cucumbers with sauerkraut kale sautéed in mounds of coconut oil leftover shredded pork sands the sauces sautéed in coconut oil until crisp with green onions. You have got to try this meal. It's delectable and perfectly balanced then about six to eight hours after that breakfast slash lunged.

Here a couple of other options to spark your meal creativity

- Arugula tossed with olive oil.
- Balsamic topped with beef.
- Pork combo burger patties with salt pepper.
- Horseradish sauerkraut sautéed with asparagus.
- A bit of carrot cooked with lard.
- Some jicama chips.

Of course, everything is drizzled with even more oil your gut is going to love you with this one now if I'm doing a carb up with this second meal. I'll want way less fat on my plate, so we'll go with something like this grass-fed bison kimchi and some greens with a bit of avocado oil apple cider vinegar maple syrup and topped with a chopped apple and some raisins this has everything you need to stay happy and satisfied. Through your carb-up, finally, if I get hungry come nighttime, I'll spring for a keto milkshake or a delicious fat bomb.

Chapter 1

How Intermittent Fasting Works?

Intermittent fasting refers to meal planning that alternates between fasting and eating periods. The purpose is to burn physically long enough to burn body fat. Although research is currently underway and this method may not be suitable for everyone. There is evidence that, when done correctly. Intermittent fasting can:

- Reduce weight.

- Reduce blood pressure.

- Reduce cholesterol.

- Control of diabetes.

- Improve brain health.

During meals, the carbohydrates in the diet are broken down into glucose. Glucose is absorbed into the bloodstream through the intestinal wall and transported to various organs, where it is an essential source of energy. Excess glucose is stored in the form of glycogen and fat for later use in the liver and adipose tissue. When the body is in a fast state between meals, the liver converts glucose back into glucose to continue supplying energy to the body.

Usually, an inactive person takes 10-12 hours to consume glycogen stores. However, anyone who exercises can do so in a short time. Once glycogen is depleted in the liver, the body is absorbed into the tissues of the body in energy deposits. When fat is broken down into free fatty acids, they are then converted into extra metabolic fuel in the liver.

In this way, if the fasting condition lasts for a long time. The body burns fat for energy and loses extra fat. Losing excess fat translates into numerous health benefits. Insulin is a hormone required to drive glucose into the cells. Insulin levels are adjusted to meet the amount of glucose in the blood, i.e., higher after meals and less between meals since insulin is empty after every meal. Insulin levels are high most of the time throughout the day.

Due to insulin anesthesia, high insulin levels can be stabilized, causing insulin anesthesia— prediction and diabetes type 2. Fasting helps to keep insulin levels low, this reduces the risk of diabetes. Fasting also has a beneficial effect on the brain. It challenges the mind in the same way that physical or cognitive exercise does. It promotes the preparation of neurotrophic factors, which support the growth and survival of neurons.

However, fasting for all. Among those who try to fast are: - Children and adolescents - Pregnant or lactating women - People with eating disorders, diabetes type 1, advanced diabetes, or some other medical problem - overweight or the weak can be fasting unsafe, or if not done correctly.

There are various approaches to fasting intermittently. But the easiest thing to achieve is probably one that only enhances your daily routine. A regular 16-hour cycle followed by an 8-hour meal window is usually lasting. From time to time, fasting to be safe and effective fast, it should be combined with balanced foods that provide proper nutrition.

Staying hydrated, and knowing your physical limits while fasting is essential. The fast should break slowly. Avoid eating unhealthy foods, especially after fasting.

What Is Intermittent Fasting?

The concept of intermittent fasting suggests that you would skip one or more meals in a row to tap into your body fat stores to burn off your body fat and to achieve a higher level of metabolic flexibility. That is, you're going to use these periods of not eating to repair your body to upregulate enzyme systems that pull the fat out of storage to build more mitochondria, which is where the fat burns.

The idea of intermittent fasting was initially more extended periods a day. At least in my estimation, 24 hours is probably the minimum of what I would call intermittent fasting. Now a lot of people are using the term intermittent fasting to apply what I would call occasional eating, which is a compressed eating window, so for instance. I generally eat from 1:30 in the afternoon until 7 p.m. I don't eat consistently to about eat two meals a day instead of three, and those are the meal times that give me 18 to 19 hours a day.

Where I'm not eating and where my body is undergoing all of these tremendous metabolic changes. I get greater metabolic flexibility greater metabolic efficiency. I'm burning off my stored body fat. I'm entering a period of what we might call a tapa G where the cells start to some housekeeping and housecleaning, all of which are contemplated to address an arena where we might be looking at longevity or more significant health or reduction of risk for certain diseases of civilization.

So, the idea of fasting intermittently again it's sort of up to the person like. I like to go at least a day without eating before. I call that intermittent fasting; otherwise, I call it a compressed eating window. The beauty of having established metabolic flexibility is that you don't suffer from skipping a meal or two or three in a row the idea is that if you're that good at taking fat out of your stored - body fat and combusting it for energy your body doesn't care where the power came from doesn't care whether it came from a plate of food or where they came from your hips or thighs.

That one of the most empowering things about this concept of metabolic flexibility is that you can go long periods without eating and have zero negative impact on your energy on your mood on your muscle mass on whether or not you get sick. Even almost no effect on your hunger, so the long answer that I just gave is it's relatively easy to do if you've established metabolic flexibility if you've done the work if you've built the metabolic machinery to access stored body fat and to burn the ketones. I think intermittent fasting works for a lot of people, some people who have medical issues and would be well-served to do this under the supervision of a trained doctor. It would be people who you know who have diabetes or women who are trying to conceive.

You know people with diagnosed diseases of certain types. Indeed, they'd be well advised to work with a physician. But otherwise, for most people, it's worth a try to you know do a foray into intermittent fasting. I don't think there's a perfect fasting window. I think it varies from individual to individual. I know some people who have breakfast and then don't eat until the next breakfast a day. Later or till lunch a day and a half later. When I fast, it's typically, I go from dinner one night to dinner the next night, and a lot of times, it's not that I planned it. It's that it just happened like I had a long day. I got involved in meetings, or I was traveling. I only didn't find time to eat. I wasn't hungry. I didn't need to eat. So, I found myself going 24 hours without eating. Typically, I stick to a regular eating schedule, which is 1:30 in the afternoon for my first meal and 7:00 7:30 at night for my second meal.

I don't have any other than the two meals a day schedule that I sort of it here too. I'm very flexible in how I skip meals the easiest way to determine. You're ready to start intermittent fasting if you wake up in the morning, and you don't need to eat or if you can skip a meal without getting hangry. You find that you have enough energy to get you to know 7, 8, 9, and 10 hours through the day without eating or a whole night of sleep. Then waking up in the morning and not eating or maybe going to the gym and doing the workout fasted and not feeling hangry or feeling like you're going to pass out from work. You did those are all indicators that you're becoming better at burning fat. You're deriving the energy from your stored body fat, and you don't require a meal to top off your energy stores.

The Fasted State

During fasting, your hormonal stimulus is glucagon. Glucagon stimulates and regulates a lot of these pathways. What I'm going to focus on today is the flux of metabolites in the fasted state. I have drawn the primary tissues that are involved in the fasting response you have the muscle the adipose tissue liver and kidney during fasting you have 18 amino acids that go through transamination and primarily produce alanine, and glutamine alanine will go to the liver.

In the liver, alanine is converted to glucose. Glucose is then used by the rest of the tissues primarily by the brain. The brain loves glucose, and so it's a huge energy sink the other essential tablets that are used for gluconeogenesis will focus here on the adipose tissue. Adipose tissue during fasting triglycerides is cleaved to free fatty acids and glycerol. The glycerol is another substrate for gluconeogenesis and produces glucose during the fasting state. The fatty acids go to the liver, and the fatty acids are used to make ketone bodies.

This process is your fatty acid oxidation or beta-oxidation. The ketone bodies are a form of energy, and the liver releases them. The liver makes ketone bodies; it does not use ketone bodies if the brain and muscle mainly use ketone bodies. We've talked about the adipose tissue. We've talked about the muscle the one amino acid that I haven't finished with yet is glutamine. Glutamine will go to the kidney, and in the kidney glutamine, the carbon backbones are used to make glucose through gluconeogenesis. But glutamine also releases ammonia. This ammonia is essential. I just told you that fatty acid is used to produce ketone bodies in the liver.

They're mild acids, so it's essential for the mild acids to be neutralized, and so the ammonia produced from tight glutamine rates. The acidity of those ketone bodies in the urine so glutamine does two things and makes glucose. It gives you vapor to titrate those ketone bodies, so in summary, then the big picture is other tissues contribute to the synthesis of glucose your muscle gives you amino acids and an amino acid alanine goes to glucose. The liver glutamine goes to glucose in the kidney the adipose tissue contributes glycerol, which is used for gluconeogenesis the free fatty acids are an essential fuel that'll go to the liver to make ketone bodies.

One important thing about the ketone bodies is that they're used in what's called fuel sparing if your body kept using those amino acids. Your muscles would be completely depleted, and the diaphragm is the most they're most susceptible to this. Therefore, the brain switches from using just glucose in prolonged fasting to using ketone bodies.

So basically, it switches from glucose to using fat because ketone bodies come from those fatty acids when it does this you need to make less glucose. Thus, gluconeogenesis decreases, and the proteolysis, the breakdown of your muscle decreases, and your body's protected as long as you have fat. You'll be excellent for a prolonged fast once you've depleted that fat. Unfortunately, you go back to using the amino acids.

Fasted and Your Metabolism

The human body has immense plasticity, the ability to adapt to unimaginable stressors to maintain homeostasis, a state of living that is no different when fasting abstaining from all nutritional energy that we receive from our macronutrients. How does it keep you alive when you do not consume food for days at a time? Does your metabolism change? How do your hormones change? I'll tell you we know that metabolism does not slow from something relatively mild like a 16-hour fast.

But after several days of no energy intake, your metabolism may decrease to compensate influenced chiefly by the decreases in leptin, which binds your hypothalamus, which controls your metabolic rate through actions like spontaneous movement. Which will reduce to pay for the lack of energy intake? As fasting continues, blood glucose sugar levels decrease before eventually leveling out. Decreases further substantiate this in glucose metabolism as the cells mostly begin to shift toward fat metabolism. Again, this is also evidenced as lipids fats are released from adipocytes fat cells to be taken up by other cells of the body and for the use in fat metabolism. Predictably ketones also increase as the liver begins converting lipids to ketones to fuel the brain and other ketone consuming cells.

Finally, many different amino acids change in concentration. But notably, leucine content skyrockets. Because of protein breakdown from degradation within the cells of the body. While I already mentioned leptin, the hormone glucagon increases, and insulin decreases as glucose decreases glucagon to stimulate gluconeogenesis, the formation of new glucose from the liver and kidneys releasing it into the bloodstream to maintain blood glucose. While insulin decreases as the pancreas does not get the stimulus to release insulin due to decrease blood glucose levels.

As a backup mechanism, cortisol also increases if the fast continues beyond several days. As cortisol further stimulates the release of a variety of substrates highest in the morning, finally, growth hormone also pulses throughout 24 hours increased at night to stimulate fat breakdown from the adipocytes. Overall you can fully expect a shift from a glucose centric metabolism to a fatter centric metabolism as a variety of hormones interplay to fulfill the overall result of keeping you alive and functional.

Fasted and Your Brain

Some of the ways the past thing can affect your brain and your mental health. I think you're going to love learning about what the brain and the nerve cells are doing for you while you fast. There are two types of intermittent fasting try fasting and water fasting with water fasting; you could drink water. But in a dry fast, staying from both food and water and it's called intermittent fasting. Because it's done at regular intervals, both types of passing have a profound effect on how your brain works and even increases the production of nerve cells, and the mind is a pretty fantastic place.

We're discovering using some pretty amazing things, one of them is that during fasting, it kicks into gear and increases the production of certain substances. One of these substances is a protein called brain-derived neurotrophic factor or BDNF. This protein helps to keep the nerve cells working and growing. But it also enhances their function. It improves brain circuitry increases the production of nerve cells that protects the brain cells from premature death. It also increases what is known as brain plasticity brain.

Plasticity is the brain's ability to create new pathways that give you many benefits, including adapting and learning needs E&M essentially helps to rewire your brain. This brain plasticity happens even at the level of the synapse.

What Is the Synapse?

A synapse is a junction between nerve cells that allows for impulses traveled from one nerve to the nest BDNF controls excitability and regulation at the synaptic level. We can modify our responses to certain stimuli. Our events started Belington, our mood, depending on the situation. We can control our feelings better by either reducing or increasing the chemical response at the level of the nerve cell to adapt to our environment.

It also helps with learning memory and focusing on a task, so what else does BDNF do it combat a process called excitotoxin city in the brain. You might have guessed excitotoxin city isn't a good thing, so what is it exciting toxicity is the process in which neurons are damaged and killed by over activation of nerve cell receptors in the brain. Under normal circumstances with healthy brain cells, chemicals known as neurotransmitters are released at the level of the synapse.

This allows impulses or information to be passed from one cell to the next exciting toxicity causes overstimulation of the neurons due to excessive release of certain chemicals, and it damages and kills your brain cells in the process. What happens when there's a reduction in the BDNF well there's a correlation between low levels of BDNF and certain diseases low levels of BDNF are associated with neurodegenerative diseases such as Parkinson's disease Alzheimer's disease multiple sclerosis and high intense illness and even depression decreased levels of BDNF also have an effect on learning, and BDNF decreases with age there are several ways to increase BDNF.

Fasted and Your Muscle Mass

I want to talk about the connection between fasting and building muscle. It's not just about the fat loss when it comes to putting on the right muscle, and it has some benefits. And I'll leave that with the study of the Western Journal of Medicine. According to this research, it was done after three days of fasting. Keep in mind that this extension is fasting, not just intermittent fasting, but whatever they found, there was a three. One hundred and fifty-five percent increase in hormones of human development is excellent. Still, a different study published in the Journal of Endocrinology Metabolism found that the human growth hormone has increased fivefold by just one hundred-day fast. Now I'm talking about this before it sounds a bit like a broken record.

I'm always referring to the human reproductive hormone when it comes to intermittent fasting. I want to do is Explain how the human growth hormone is like the effect when it comes down to building muscle, you see that the human growth hormone is just Not random, it is a 191 amino chain, which means that it acts like a protein in the body that moves around it and now stimulates the development of different things.

The soma in the pituitary gland is generated by the cells and what chondrocyte cells say they are divided into the cartilage. Now you will be surprised what you have to do with the cartilage of the muscle. When these cells divide, they become dynamic. Collagen Synthesis and Collagen Production Collagen give structure to our cells when it comes to muscle. Well, the muscles help in growth and formation, but collagen is also going to help us do many other things like tendon.

In the power of this and everything like that, you may have noticed by now that anyone who goes to human growth hormone therapy or any type of anti-aging treatment usually ends up with good skin, which is why it's just the reason is that they have increased collagen production and collagen is also helpful in helping your skin, but when human pro-tan's down to protein. It does something special when you see that it has low protein oxidation.

So, we have two different things:

- Protein synthesis.
- Protein oxidation.

Where you are eating more protein, they are oxidized and eventually toxic, and then we have protein synthesis, which reduces the rate of protein oxidation in the human growth hormone formulation, which means you consume more protein are used. Therefore, when you are fasting, the human growth hormone increases five times. NG can be mighty when it comes to muscle building. Now let's talk about son hydroxybutyrate. I have spoken about beta-hydroxybutyrate when it comes to ketosis, but I don't always mention it when it comes to fasting you see when you go into fasting your body uses this ketone body. It manufactures what is called beta-hydroxybutyrate.

Now, beta-hydroxybutyrate does many things inside the body. But in this particular case, I want to talk about research that looked at players who were already in a ketogenic or fast-growing state of son hydroxy biotite, and their muscles when they were working. How did they affect the surface, did they see the athletes that had to work with while fasting, but they measured their son's hydroxybutyrate levels?

But then they measured their muscle cells. Take a look at some of the things they learned that the presence of hydroxybutyrate on their muscles increased the survival rate of cells means that you didn't burn muscle tissue every time you exercised while you were working if you smoked a little flesh. So, if the son hydroxy biotite, which is the result of fasting, helps the muscles to survive, that is a good thing. Still, the other thing that happened with this son hydroxy biotite was that he found in mitochondria—increased ATP function. This means that physically eating your muscles yes by eating and not working out. Also, given the increase is such amazing right muscle. If you hear about the meditation, then you are a limiting factor in muscle building if you have never seen these Belgian blue cows before with cows that are wholly united with their brains.

They look weird so that they can make genetic changes. Deficiency of myostatin means that their muscle is capable of growing in a high amount. There is a high level of myostatin in humans. Myostatin prevents our muscles from eventually increasing and the way it works, which is known as the auto cream function. Muscle cells are never found to be primarily blocked or eventually enlarged so that more and more mutation becomes less muscular and more muscular. There is a very complicated relationship. There was a study that looked at it, and the International Journal of Sports and Health found that test subjects who exposed to only a small amount of testosterone are on a large scale.

The significant decrease in their levels of metastases in many muscles means that it can only be used in certain parts of the body. I was not systemic. A slight increase in testosterone equals less somatostatin, which means that your body can exert as much muscle as you were genetically capable of before testosterone. But now we have to create a link between fasting and testosterone so that you can see the endocrinology of the European Journal that I have given a lot of references to. Studies have shown that fasting increases what is known as luteinizing hormone.

The luteinizing hormone is secreted by the pituitary gland, which ultimately produces more testosterone and equals more testosterone to latex cells. This is the first step in the equation. So, fasting is high. Increase testosterone by one hundred and eighty percent, and if we have an increase in testosterone, then we have a decrease in myostatin. And we're able to feel a lot better in the process So that you have a combination of human growth hormone metastatic and, of course, a beta-hydroxybutyrate, which is safe, puts you at a triple risk when it comes to being able to build muscle to protect your muscles.

Chapter 2

What is Intermittent Fasting and Why Would You Do It?

What is intermittent fasting?

Intermittent fasting refers to maintaining zero or very low-calorie intake periodically for a specified period. Cyclical means not always fasting. It can be one day a week or one day a month, but not for several days. This is very different from the traditional method of digging the valley or losing weight. Intermittent fasting generally means not eating for 18-36 hours.

Zero-calorie or very low-calorie intake is also different from the traditional Pigu. Some people who eat grains can eat fruits and vegetables, but intermittent fasting does not eat anything except drinking water and supplementing vitamins and electrolytes.

Many people feel a little scared when they hear about fasting. In fact, in ancient times and famines, people often ate up and down, often in intermittent fasting. High blood pressure and diabetes at that time were rare and not entirely accidental. Also, we often inadvertently fast intermittently in our daily life, but we do not pay attention to. For example, after dinner at six, sleep on an empty stomach at night, and sometimes some people do not eat breakfast until noon the next day fasting for 18 hours. Furthermore, sometimes we are busy with work and can't afford to eat. This is also intermittent fasting.

How to Perform Intermittent Fasting?

Intermittent fasting every day, for example: only eat between noon and 6 pm; eat three meals early in the morning and then fast from 6 p.m. to 7 a.m., or eat only twice a day as needed. Intermittent fasting every week, for example: fasting every other day, or 5: 2 (five days to eat regularly, choose two days to fast).

Intermittent fasting every month, for example, five days a month.

What Are the Benefits of Intermittent Fasting in Weight Loss?

- Reduce the risk of cardiovascular system disease and diabetes.
- Promote the body to use fat as an energy source to achieve the effect of weight loss.
- Significantly increase growth hormone secretion and promote metabolism.

Why Is Intermittent Fasting So Popular?

Intermittent fasting (from now on referred to as IF) is very popular in Europe and the United States and has multiple benefits to the body, such as increasing muscle and fat, improving immunity, helping the body detox, and even prolonging life.

Fasting is very natural. In primitive society, we often had to be hungry for a long time to eat the next meal. When you are sick, your appetite will be reduced, and your body is telling you to use fasting to speed up recovery.

The most common and feasible fasting method is too fast for 16 hours (including sleep time) and eats 8 hours (usually two meals). During the 16 hours of fasting, you can only drink water, tea, or pure coffee. For example, you eat dinner at 6 p.m., go to bed at 10 a.m., get up at 6 a.m. without breakfast, you have to wait at least 10 a.m. before you can start to eat, and you can eat at will during the 8 hours from 10 a.m. to 6 p.m. (Of course recommend healthy food).

A survey by the International Food Information Council Foundation found that intermittent fasting was the most popular dieting method last year. Recently, Jack Dorsey, the president of Twitter, claimed that he only eats one meal a day, causing a lot of attention on social media. Many people criticize this approach as being too extreme, but it is undeniable that this is the current trend.

Impact on Health

The human evidence for —intermittent fasting‖ is still weak, but more and more studies have found improvements in different health indicators in addition to weight, especially blood lipids. Besides, those studies also mentioned that —intermittent fasting‖ may have more unique metabolic benefits than eating less frequently.

The most impressive and most controversial of these health benefits is longevity. Fasting can restart some regeneration processes in the human body, and prolonging life by limiting calories has been demonstrated in some animal models, but not all. But keep in mind that those animals spend most of their lives either on a low-calorie diet or intermittent fasting. It is not known whether —intermittent fasting‖ can delay human life. Even if it can, which variant is most effective, it will take weeks, months, or years to make a big difference.

Assessing the potential metabolic benefits of -intermittent fasting‖ is a long-term process. As mentioned in a 2015 systematic literature review, preliminary evidence is promising, but strong evidence remains few, so more human research is needed before fasting recommendations are a health intervention.

What Happens to Your Body When You Have Fast 16 Hours?

Fasting is a new tendency in modern society. Every religion has a fasting rule because we believe that fasting encourages us to be able to pray and be closer to God. We develop the ability to focus on God through fasting, and therefore we experience deep spiritual insight. But the modern concept of fasting shows us that, because of the mental benefits, fasting can be useful to achieve the goal of health.

What Is the Post?

Fasting is a must in every religion. For example, in Islam during the Ramadan month and in many religious communities, such as Buddhist monks and nuns, who follow the rules of Vinaya and do partial fasting. This is the process by which an individual eagerly limits the intake of food or drink. According to medicine, starvation means an empty stomach for a couple of hours or after the complete digestion of one meal.

However, fasting is a method without food, including religious rituals, detoxification, cleansing of the stomach, etc.

What Happens to Your Body: Day 1-2 Energy Lose?

At the cellular level, several things happen that cause hunger and fatigue in this first step. When you eat regularly, your body breaks down glucose to get the energy necessary for normal functioning. While you are fasting, your body needs to produce sugar to generate electricity, so a process called gluconeogenesis begins. During gluconeogenesis, your liver converts non-carbohydrate substances, such as lactate, amino acids, and fats, into glucose. As your body goes into Battery Saver mode, your basal metabolic rate, or BMR, becomes more efficient and uses less energy. This energy-saving process includes lowering your heart rate and blood pressure. At this point, you may feel exhausted. However, if you last a little longer, part of this lost energy will return.

What Happens to Your Body: Day 3-7 Fat Burning Regimen?

When you consume a typical carbohydrate-rich diet, your body breaks down sugar and turns starch into glucose. Glucose is the primary source of energy for our bodies. However, when you fast or begin to suffer from ketosis, glucose levels become limited, and your body must turn to fat stores to get the energy it needs. Your body breaks down fat into glycerin and fatty acids. The liver synthesizes ketones using glycerol. Glycerin is broken down by the liver to get extra glucose, and finally, these ketones are used by your brain as glucose becomes less available.

What Happens to Your Body: Day 8-15 Healing Mode?

In the third stage, your body begins to go into a —healing mode.‖ This healing process begins when your digestive system rests from the everyday stressors and toxins that it carries daily. As a result, less free radical enters your body, and oxidative stress decreases. On the other hand, fasting causes stress, which provides additional benefits. This kind of mild stress is comparable to the stress caused by exercise, which ultimately makes you stronger, and your immune system more stable.

The Benefits of Fasting: What Happens to Your Body When We Fast?

1. Fasting Improves Brain Activity

Many might think that this is a little strange, but fasting indeed speeds up the brain. Studies have shown that in the event of starvation, the energy of the human brain increases because it changes the specific functions of the cells and, at the same time, increases the production of the protein, which is responsible for the activation of brain stem cells to activate new neurons. It also protects brain cells to go through the changes that occur in Parkinson's and Alzheimer's.

2. Improves Peace of Mind and Spiritualism

When we talk about human well-being, we cover not only physical health but also mental health, because a healthy body and a healthy mind are the two main assets of any person to control the overall function of life. Fasting for religious rituals makes us experience joy and mental satisfaction, as it helps us approach the Almighty. To achieve this, we deprive ourselves of the comfort that gives clarity to our thoughts. Therefore, fasting is necessary to purify our souls.

3. Helps Regulate Eating Habits

The modern lifestyle has changed all areas, especially our eating habits. Many are addicted to fast foods that are readily available everywhere, and for this reason, they face stomach and digestive problems. Fasting is an age-old practice that helps to start a healthy eating habit in everything. Five to six hours of fasting between meals or intermittent fasting reduces the consumption of junk food and indirectly supports the digestive system to work efficiently.

4. Helps Detoxify the Body

The term —detoxification‖ means a lot that relates to our well-being. This is perhaps one of the most amazing benefits of the post, which directly improves our system. During fasting, the lack of food for an extended period lays glycogen, which was stored by the liver in the form of glucose. Our body begins to decompose fat and release accumulated harmful chemicals from fats into the body and thus eliminate them with the help of the kidneys, lungs, lymph nodes, and skin.

5. Helps with Weight Loss

I am sure that with the help of fasting, anyone can lose weight naturally without spending hours on training. Intermittent fasting or random fasting for several hours a day eliminates fat cells from burning for energy. However, those who are overweight adhere to a strict dietary rule, ignoring tasty food for a long time, but this only deprives them of a lot. People can eat at regular intervals of 5-6 hours, and they will follow fasting for the remaining hours. A few low-calorie foods will prove more effective. Fasting is a new tendency in modern society. Every religion has a fasting rule because we believe that fasting encourages us to be able to pray and be closer to God. We develop the ability to focus on God through fasting, and therefore we experience deep spiritual insight. But the modern concept of fasting shows us that, because of the mental benefits, fasting can be useful to achieve the goal of health.

Can You Lose Weight Eating 2 Meals A Day?

We are often told that skipping one of the three meals of the day does not work. But it is quite possible to lose weight by taking only two meals a day without endangering your health. Sometimes we think we take three meals a day when this is not necessarily the case. A cup of tea, a glass of fruit juice, a simple yogurt, or even a quick toast is not considered a real meal.

To slim down with only two meals a day, you can skip breakfast or dinner but never lunch. This is intermittent fasting. It is not a diet, but a food habit that you give to your body. In the beginning, you can start with one day a week, then two, and so on so as not to rush your body. You have the choice between eating only morning and noon or only lunch and dinner.

Important

If you want to lose weight, eat three meals normally. It is best to eat less (fruit, vegetables, rice soup) or not to eat dinner, especially after 8 p.m., you can't eat anything, and don't eat it.

Or if you eat two meals a day, breakfast and lunch, replace fruit with dinner. Although this method works, you must take good results when you see results (if your body shape has reached your expected goals). The rest of the time is to pay attention to diet, cannot eat anything oily.

Then teach you the cruelest trick, do not eat meat, eat three meals a day full of seven (after 8 p.m., you cannot eat anything, do not eat). It won't take long for you to lose weight. However, this method is recommended for fat people. If you want to stay in shape, you don't have to use it so hard.

Eating two meals a day may seem crazy to you, even impossible or too difficult to follow. It is not only possible, but it is also how we ate before. This is no longer the case today, but the first men spent their day looking for food, eating a big meal in the evening, and they certainly had no obesity problems.

You may have heard the term intermittent fasting. It is a way of describing the diets which oscillate between periods of feeding and periods of starvation. Eating one meal a day is considered a strict time-limited form of eating since most of the day is spent fasting.

How Can Just Two Meal a Day Help You Be Healthy?

The idea behind eating just one meal a day is to eat less simply. Once the body adjusts to eating only once a day, it turns your stored fat into fuel, and ultimately you lose weight and become less hungry.

Ashley Smith, a nutrition therapy practitioner in Berkeley, explains, ―You can become more effective mentally and physically.‖ ―It may take a few weeks to go from‖ sugar burner ―to‖ fat burner, ―but that will be done, especially when consuming a wide variety of high-quality fats, whole / nutritious vegetables, and good quality meat.‖

The secret is to eat a very nutritious meal and eat until you are full. You can choose the time of day, but it's easier to eat at the end of the day. Most people lose weight with this diet without having to watch their portion sizes or count calories.

Can I Lose Weight by Eating Two Meals a Day?

Some diets claim that eating up to six meals a day boosts your metabolism and keeps you from being hungry. The only problem is that regularly eating throughout the day encourages an obsession with food and overconsumption.

It also makes it easier to exceed your daily calorie limits. The truth is that eating six meals a day doesn't have a significant impact on your metabolism. You're just going to burn ten more calories. Some experts claim that not eating for a while slows metabolism. And that's true. But it would take three days of fasting to have a noticeable impact on your metabolism.

It seems that the more you eat, the more you want to eat. Everyone knows that. This leads to an obsession with food and overconsumption. The opposite effect also occurs. The less you eat, the less you want to eat.

When you are trying to lose or maintain your weight, it is easier to lose weight by eating less often. Ultimately, eating six meals a day makes you want to eat more and more often.

It is not for everyone. Not everyone will be satisfied with just one meal a day. Some people prefer to distribute their nutritional intake throughout the day. Eating 2 to 3 meals a day will always bring the same benefits.

Some nutritionists warn against restricting food to one meal a day and remind that it can promote an unhealthy relationship with food.

Some nutritionists claim that restricting meals once a day can encourage an obsession with food. While this may be true for some, many people who have adopted this lifestyle notice a significant decrease in hunger and a healthier relationship with food.

What Are the Side Effects of Intermittent Fasting?

Intermittent fasting is gaining popularity, and many people hope to lose weight in this way. Why can it help lose weight? What risks might you face? -Live well,‖ ask nutritionists to analyze. However, to date, studies on intermittent fasting have been small and short-term. The sustainability and safety of intermittent fasting are currently limited to six months.

It should be reminded that although intermittent fasting can reduce weight in some people, it is not a panacea for improving health. If you overeat or eat unhealthy foods during non-fasting periods, you will not lose weight.

Another risk is inadequate intake of vitamins and minerals, which can affect normal cell function, growth, etc. If you choose to implement this diet therapy, it is recommended that you pay attention to food choices when you are not fasting. You should eat nutritious, high fiber, low fat and sugar, and balanced food.

1. Hunger

If you usually eat 5-6 times a day, the body will expect food at the times you typically use it to eat. According to Stephanie, the presence of the hormone glycerin is responsible for hunger.

Usually, hunger peaks at breakfast, lunch, and dinner and is partly regulated by food intake. When you first start the fasting diet, glycerin levels will continue to increase, so you feel hungry.

—During the initial 3-5 days, it will feel awful, but there will be times where you reach the dining window and no longer feel hungry,‖ Stephanie said.

Specialist in nutrition and weight loss as well as a certified cardiologist, Dr. Luiza Petre, advises beginners on a fasting diet to fight hunger in the first 1-2 weeks by drinking plenty of water.

It aims to make the stomach feel full, make us stay awake, and get used to putting something in the mouth. Within 30 minutes of waking up, at least drink about 250 ml of water. When hungry, drink another 250 ml. What the fasting diet will teach you is that what you think hunger is thirst or boredom. Drinking black coffee and tea can also overcome desire.

Besides, sufficient sleep needs, stay busy, and avoid strenuous exercise in the first few weeks, because these activities will increase hunger. Eat enough the previous day and eat enough carbohydrates, healthy fats, and protein.

2. Headaches

Because the body is getting used to a new eating schedule, headaches are widespread. Edward Vasquez, a YouTuber who talks a lot about fasting through his Fledge Fitness account, provides tips for running it.

According to him, dehydration is one of the main factors. So, make sure you drink lots of water during fasting and meal times. According to Stephanie, headaches can also be caused by decreased blood sugar levels, and stress hormones released by the brain when fasting.

Over time, the body will get used to the new eating schedule. However, you try to be free from stress.

3. Lack of Energy

As a result of previously, you are accustomed to eating all day; your body may feel weak and underpowered because the body no longer gets constant fuel intake. Make sure you don't do many activities that consume too much energy, especially in the early weeks.

For example, avoid strenuous exercise and replace it with walking or yoga. Then, sleeping longer is also quite helpful.

4. Burning, Bloating and Constipation

The stomach will produce acids to help digest food. So, when we don't eat, we can feel like a burning sensation in the body. This can occur in the form of the discomfort of moderate-intensity throughout the day. This feeling will disappear over time.

So, keep consuming water, support our body to sleep, and avoid greasy and spicy foods because it can worsen the burning sensation. If the burning feels increasingly uncomfortable, consult a doctor.

Fasting diets can also cause constipation or constipation if the body is not hydrated enough so that it will cause bloating and discomfort. Stephanie suggests drinking plenty of water to overcome these problems and can prevent headaches and make the body more energized.

5. Feel Cold

The tips of the toes and hands that are cold when fasting are common but positive. When fasting, blood flow increases to fat reserves or adipose tissue. This can help move fat to the muscles, which means it can be burned as a fuel for power.

Stephanie said the condition of decreased blood sugar would also make us more sensitive and more comfortable to feel cold. Fight the cold feeling by drinking tea, taking warm baths, using layered clothing, and avoiding being outdoors when it's cold for a long time.

6. Overeating

People who are new to the fasting diet will tend to overeat. This could be because they thought that the calorie size did not affect or because they were starving, so they were very excited to meet food.

Planning food to be consumed can help you maintain ideal food portions. —When the fasting period is over, we must be careful with eating portions. You may indeed feel like eating everything, but choose healthy food options,‖ Stephanie said.

Note these symptoms usually only occur during the week or a maximum of the initial three weeks. To avoid this, you can do it gradually so that the fasting diet will feel natural and healthy. So that appetite decreases mental acuity increases, then waist circumference decreases.

Fasting diets are also not intended for everyone—for example, diabetics, pregnant women, nursing mothers, or children. People who have chronic diseases also need to see a doctor first before starting a fasting diet.

People who have a history of risk of eating disorders also need to avoid fasting in various forms. There are times when the side effects of the fasting diet should not be ignored.

Chapter 3

Women's and Men's Guide to Intermittent Fasting

Discontinuous fasting may be an eating wherein you abandon food for a selected measure of your time a day. To help you explore your day, here's a manual for a way to plan your dinners during discontinuous fasting. What's more, recollect: Although this eating plan is organized around once you eat, what you eat is so far significant. During the timeframes, when you're eating, you will need to consider solid fats, clean protein, and sugars from whole food sources. While fasting is often overpowering, particularly on the off chance that you haven't done it previously, irregular fasting can be significantly simpler than numerous different types of eating plans.

When you start your irregular fasting venture, you'll find that you feel more full and may keep the dinners you are doing eat basically. There are a few varied ways you'll quickly, so I separated all of the various plans beneath into apprentice, moderate, and progressed alongside a commonplace supper plan for each day. The blend of supplements will offer you the vitality you've got to enhance the benefits of your fasting venture. Make some extent to think about a person's food bigotries, and utilize this as a guide for your specific wellbeing case, and alter from that time.

Keep in mind; discontinuous fasting doesn't mean calorie-controlled, so make sure to eat as per your own caloric needs. If you're a novice, start by just eating between the long stretches of 8 a.m. also, 6 p.m. is a fantastic method to plunge your toes into the fasting waters. This arrangement permits you to eat each feast additionally to some the thought of irregular fasting is entirely not something for the foremost part recommended for end of the day weight reduction. As indicated by Michael Wosley, restorative columnist and creator of The Fast Diet, he was initially suspicious of the technique, as well.

Nonetheless, following a time of research and playing guinea pig together with his eating routine, Wosley lost around 9 kg and a fourth of his muscle to fat ratio and has since been spruiking the benefits of fasting. A day of fasting may include something just like the accompanying: for breakfast, a dish (before the toast), berries and a tablespoon of yogurt, or ¼ cup heated beans on toast. Lunch could incorporate a touch plate of mixed greens with fish, egg or grains, and dinner could be something sort of a little pan-fried food, salmon and vegetables, or another serving of mixed greens.

It unquestionably sounds feasible; be that because it may, nibbling within the middle of dinners would presumably set you over as far as possible, so just in case you are a nibbler, it'd be increasingly troublesome. Wosley himself deals together with his fasting days by having a 300 Calorie breakfast at 7 a.m. (300 Calories being what could be compared to 2 cuts of light bread and a couple of boiled eggs), and afterward not eating again until his 300 Calorie dinner at 7 p.m.! Merely the thought of going 10 hours without eating makes my head turn, primarily as going this point allotment without fuel makes bound to cause a make a plunge glucose levels, bringing about that trademark shakes, even as an extreme diminishing focused and mental sharpness. Snacks yet at an equivalent time get in 14 hours of fasting inside a 24-hour term.

12 Health Benefits of Intermittent Fasting

1. May Bolster Sound Weight the Board

Via preparing your body to consume fat for vitality, discontinuous fasting can cash in of your body's regular weight reduction components. Additionally, the effortlessness of the arrangement implies you're substantially more susceptible to stick with it! At the purpose, once you practice discontinuous fasting and effectively switch your body into the fat-copying mode, your body is utilizing adrenaline to discharge put away glycogen and access fat to repeat. These expanded adrenaline levels can assist with boosting your digestion.

2. May Help Your Vitality

Not in the least like such vast numbers of calorie limitation eats less, which will cause you to feel lazy, the irregular fasting plan is meant to assist stable hormone levels with the goal that you're in every case effectively going to put away fat for vitality.

3. May Advance Mental Lucidity and Core Interest

Irregular fasting can help your intellectual competence since it expands your BDNF, which supports cerebrum network and new neuron development.

4. May Bolster Psychological Capacity

The hormonal changes that happen once you follow irregular fasting have been seemed to help memory and cerebrum work.

5. May Help Continue Solid Glucose Levels

Fasting can help bolster the support of typical glucose levels. While you're in your fasting window, no new glucose is being provided to your body, which means your organization must choose the choice to travel through put away glucose.

6. May Bolster Heart Wellbeing

Discontinuous fasting is an astounding supporter of heart wellbeing, in sight of its capacity to assist your liver's cholesterol creation at a substantial level.

7. May Bolster the Body's Calming Reaction

Your body depends on a procedure called ―autophagy‖ to urge out old and harmed tissues and cells. At the purpose, once you quick and offer your body a reprieve from the consistent exertion of processing food, it's by all accounts able to concentrate more vitality on typical fix endeavors, which suggests supporting your body's natural mitigating reaction. Tons of research has been embraced on the impacts of fasting during the traditional Muslim month of Ramadan, wherein starvation happens among dawn and dusk.

One such investigation, which checked fifty people getting to initiate Ramadan fasting, included estimating the degrees of fiery master cytokines in their blood. Cytokines are particles coursing within the blood that react to changes within the host's wellbeing status. They could be genius incendiary, and enhance the side effects of constant sickness – as an example, interleukin 1 (IL-1), and tumor putrefaction factor (TNF) – or mitigating, and work to decrease irritation, and return the body to a solid-state.

During the fasting time of Ramadan, the members demonstrated diminished degrees of provocative expert cytokines within the blood, alongside diminished pulse, weight, and muscle versus fat ratio. These all expanded once typical eating was continued. Another fascinating finding was that immune cells were altogether brought down during fasting, anyway, because the proposed diet recommends just two days of irregular fasting. It's suspicious that insusceptibility would be smothered end of the day.

Another vital investigation looked to research the viability of irregular vitality limitation (same standards because the 5:2 eating regimen), with constant vitality limitation, during which lower calories were devoured a day. An aggregate of 107 moderately aged ladies was partitioned into the 2 test gatherings. Through the span of a half year, they were checked for changes in weight, alongside numerous different markers of wellbeing status. His investigation uncovered comparable outcomes for every gathering, with the two eating regimens prompting weight reduction, improved insulin affectability, and diminished cholesterol and circulatory strain.

These discoveries recommend that discontinuous fasting is often looked on as an appropriate option to full-time eating less food, unquestionably an alluring alternative for those not focused on going the whole hoard. One impediment to the investigation is that because it may, was that each member was urged to eat as indicated by a Mediterranean-style diet, which is synonymous with acceptable wellbeing with its accentuation on tons of plant foods and limited quantities of meat and dairy.

Food partition records, dinner plans, and plans were provided, which can well have driven members to receive an eating regimen ton more beneficial than their standard. Such an adjustment in eating examples may need improved their outcomes more so than the structure of diet they were embraced. Do you get suspicious once you hear people raving about another eating routine that creates weight reduction simple? We do not accuse you—body synthesis will generally be drunker than the consuming fewer calories industry leads on. In an industry loaded with contrivances and trends, there's one arrangement rapidly ascending to the bleeding edge since it's the heaviness of proof behind it.

An irregular fasting diet is progressively being lauded as an eating design that advances healthy weight the board while additionally being anything, but difficult to follow. Numerous people swear it is the most integral asset they've found for weight control, and they are not envisioning things. Irregular fasting's mystery lies within the way that it moves your body from consuming carbs and sugar for fuel to consuming fat. A recent report exhibited that this arrangement could help diminish your weight by 3-8% in 3-24 weeks! We've recognized a few key reasons concerning why discontinuous fasting for weight reduction works so well.

8. Clear-cut Advantage for Managing Cravings

Taking under consideration that the minor word –fasting‖ can cause us to feel hungry, it is lovely amazement for a few discontinuous fasting adherents to seek out that, after around 1-2 weeks, they nevermore experience many cravings for food during their fasting windows. Furthermore, no, it isn't only a stunt of the psyche or extraordinary resolution. There is a logical motivation behind why this happens. One of the foremost significant impacts that discontinuous fasting has on your body is that it underpins stable glucose levels. Normal glucose levels mean fewer sugar desires.

The other cool thing that happens once you start discontinuous fasting is that it underpins substantial degrees of a hormone called -ghrelin.‖ Ghrelin is understood because of the yearning hormone. At the purpose when it's askew, that's the purpose at which you are feeling hungry constantly. Following two or three weeks of irregular fasting and stable ghrelin levels, you'll begin to ascertain decreased food cravings.

9. Common Calorie Restriction, But Better

At the bottom of just about every eating routine known to man is the idea of calorie limitation. We've all observed the recipe: Calories are eaten < calories consumed = weight reduction Calorie limitation is likewise the first motivation behind why most weight control plans flop over the end of the day. It conflicts with human instinct, and along these lines is fantastically hard to support. Irregular fasting has earned massive applause by the way that it usually prompts calorie limitation, without feeling like that's what you're doing. We wish to call it ―slippery‖ calorie limitation. Here's the reason: a run of the mill discontinuous fasting plan (eating just among early afternoon and 8:00 p.m). typically compares to skipping breakfast. Since it's hard to dine in more than a selected number of calories per feast, cutting your day from 3 dinners right down to 2 can have a noticeable impact after a while.

Studies are finished watching a gathering of individuals who were approached to confine their calories throughout the day, and another collection that was approached to follow an irregular fasting plan. Both groups determined comparative medical advantages, except the discontinuous fasting bunch, experienced progressively bolstered glucose levels. In particular, the illegal fasting bunch discovered their eating regimen significantly more sensible. For the higher a part of us, it's mentally and naturally simpler to limit our eating to a selected period, rather than to confine our general day by day caloric admission.

10. Hold Lean Muscle Mass

Maybe the best drawback of the many confined calorie abstains from food is that they need to have been demonstrated to prompt loss of slender bulk, which hinders your digestion. This is often downright terrible news for your capacity to stay up any weight reduction.

The uplifting news? Research has indicated that irregular fasting causes you to hold fit bulk while so far shedding pounds. Phew!

11. Better Eating Habits

At the purpose, once you irregular quick, you will be adhering to a littler eating window than you presumably won't. This may typically eliminate late-evening eating, which is often a shrouded culprit of overabundance calories and subtle weight gain. At the purpose, once you realize that yielding to the munchies is just getting to show yourself out of fat-consuming mode, it is a lot simpler to oppose that late-night cooler attack!

12. It's Sustainable

Maybe the most striking aspect concerning the discontinuous fasting —fever‖ is that folks are treating it less sort of an eating routine and progressively like a way of life. Such vast numbers of adherents get themselves getting healthier, yet feeling much improved and wanting to stick with this eating plan. So discontinuous fasting can immediately become how of life change, rather than an accident diet.

Chapter 4

Styles of Intermittent Fasting

What Does "Healthy" Mean to You?

For me, being healthy methods having the option to do the things you love while you feel your best. So, wellbeing for you is characterized by having the opportunity to do the things you love. What do you like to do, and how does that work with your method for eating? I love being dynamic, regardless of whether that is through a turn or lifting loads or having the option to travel. I need the opportunity to do each one of those things without feeling like my wellbeing or my body keeps me away from taking a stab at something I might want to attempt. Presently, I've generally been moderately healthy; however, I believe that irregular fasting has helped me improve my decisions. At the point when I feast prep, I consider lunch and supper and perhaps a bite. I don't stress over breakfast or heft around a ton for a day of eating. In actuality, it's only one colossal holder.

What Eating Style Encourages You to Feel You're Most Advantageous?

I have joined a few eating styles. I began discontinuous fasting, Paleo, eating less gluten, eating more vegetables, and supper preparing in 2015. I found Whole30 in 2019, and I, at present, do a blend of the entirety of the above in my way of life. Whole30 and discontinuous fasting have most affected my healthy dietary patterns.

I regularly begin to eat around 11 a.m. or then again at noon, contingent upon my lunch plan at work. I have a generous lunch, and I'm commonly not ravenous until supper. I eat at around 7 p.m. I quit eating around 8 p.m. or, on the other hand, at 9 p.m. That is a 14-to 16-hour fasting window. In the early morning, I drink dark espresso and water, and that is it.

Generally, I'm still Paleo. Discontinuous fasting permits me to be somewhat more adaptable to what I eat and when I eat. I feel my best when I'm eating in a Paleo and Whole30 way (which, for me, implies, I limit my admission of handled nourishment).

What Were Your Objectives When You Rolled Out These Improvements?

I needed to have more vitality, improve my enthusiastic wellbeing, and feel less tired by and large. I needed to settle on eating and drinking decisions dependent on how this would fuel my body, brain, and soul as opposed to considering nourishment to be either positive or negative.

Did You Beforehand Consider Nourishment to be Nourishment Decisions as Either Positive or Negative?

Indeed, particularly toward the start of finding out about sugar, gluten, and dairy. I figured it was all bad, and all needed to be avoided. Presently I don't expand these fixings to such an extent, but not because that I consider them to be terrible; they don't cause me actually to feel so incredible. It's a slight move. It's generally about how I would feel right if I don't eat this or do eat that.

Everything being equal, I'll eat high-quality pasta and, I'm alright with feeling sluggish for the remainder of the day; however, I don't consider that to be as fortunate or unfortunate. It's precisely what's beneficial to me and how it will influence me generally speaking. Another model is I will have a go at everything when I travel. That is encouraging my passionate wellbeing and my social wellbeing and takes need over clean eating regularly.

16/8 Method

It is not a diet; it is a type of intermittent fasting or time-restricted eating. During this, you can't only eat low calories food, but you can also eat a variety of food in this you spend 16 hours of each day consuming nothing but unsweetened beverages like water, coffee, and tea. But remaining 8, you are allowed to eat anything by doing this. You can get many benefits like you can lose your belly fat and get smarter.

Do You Have to Do 16/8 Every Day?

We should try this method every day because it's beneficial for us.

Is It Helpful or Not?

Helpful fasting generally includes abandoning nourishment for a few days. On account of discontinuous fasting, then again, taking regular breaks from eating is adequate. However, is this methodology compelling regarding the members' weight and digestion? What's more, what does science need to state about it? For numerous individuals, another year commonly implies making goals.

Getting thinner is one of the most critical objectives, and there's no deficiency of chances to do as such, as counting calories methodologies flourish. Be that as it may, these frequently call for surrendering specific sorts of nourishment, a methodology that is unreasonable for some over the long haul. Interim fasting speaks to an alternate method for handling muscle versus fat. It's unique about slimming down in that it doesn't concentrate on changing what you eat, but instead basically deferring when you eat and are taking longer, regular breaks from eating.

Anna Engler found this pattern for herself and has just shed more than 30 pounds. She has been fasting utilizing the 16:8 techniques for a year now, which includes abandoning potent nourishment for 16 hours while drinking just dark espresso, tea, and water. Eating is permitted during the remaining eight hours of the day. ‒I don't need to skip pizza or Turkish fringes, which are my top picks,‖ says the Berlin occupant. Engler enjoys a reprieve from eating beginning at dinnertime until lunch the next day. She says she discovers this mood to keep up, as she never especially enjoyed having breakfast in any case.

For a long time, Engler struggled with low motivation, a lack of discipline, and excessive weight. The 32 years old was significantly overweight but did not have any appetite for diets. ‒I always thought‖ they were pointless because you gain back anything you have lost right away,‖ she says. ‒This seems to be a method that is relatively easy to integrate into your day to day life without causing a lot of upheavals,‖ Says Stephen Herzing. He heads up the institute for diabetes and cancer at the Zentrum vision, and he and his team conduct research into the ways that overnight fasting affects metabolism interval fasting have many other positive effects in addition to helping people lose weight. It also makes insulin more useful again,

For example, moreover, it lowers blood pressure and prevents cardiovascular disease over the long-term, and also supports cancer treatment. Together with his team, the researcher is currently exploring the questions of how fasting can be used for therapy purposes and how drugs that imitate fasting can be developed.

5/2 method

What is the 5/2 method?

It is a type of fasting in which we eat about 25% of our total calories that are required for our bodies. Usually, we needed almost 2000 2100 calories for two days, but in this, we only consume 500 to 600 calories. When we consume low calories, it helps to reduce our weight.

How Does It Work?

I am beginning the 5:2 Diet to shed a couple of pounds. We found out about it from my better half's sister, who shed more than 20 pounds in only a few months, so my significant other chose to check it out. I'm not a colossal fanatic of diets. I believe it's increasingly about –eating less and practicing more, yet that doesn't appear to be working, so I wouldn't fret taking a stab at something new.

Like a decent spouse, when my significant other beginnings an eating routine, I attempt it to check whether it can work for me. Makes feast arranging a lot simpler. So, as I'm expounding on this moderately new eating regimen, I'm somewhat eager since today is one of my two low-calorie consumption days.

Fundamentally, the 5:2 Diet lets you eat like you regularly accomplish for five days per week; however, then eat a low, low-calorie diet (nearly fasting) on the other two days. For my significant other, this implies only 500 calories for her and 600 calories for me. I'll get into the fundamental reasons in a minute; however, you can peruse Gina Crawford's book (and it will take you around 30 minutes).

Who Found It?

As indicated by Gina Crawford, Dr. Michael Mosley is the –organizer of the 5:2 Diet and creator of The Fast Diet that I'm speculating broadly expounds than Ms. Crawford's guide for amateurs. Conceived in India, Dr. Mosley is currently a BBC TV columnist who produces appears on medicine and science.

After a short financial vocation, Mosley chose to turn into a specialist and learned at the Royal Free Hospital Medical School. Directly after he moved on from therapeutic school in 1985, he turned into an associate maker student for the BBC. It was in 2012 that he was credited with advancing the 5:2 Diet.

14/10 Method

14:10 requires you to fast for 14 hours and eat all your calories within 10 hours each day.

What happens when you don't eat for 14 hours?

During a 14-hour fast, you can expand without calorie refreshments. At the point when the 14-hour time frame is finished, you can continue your regular admission of nourishment until the following fast.

Notwithstanding weight misfortune, irregular fasting can positively affect your digestion, support cardiovascular wellbeing, and that's only the tip of the iceberg. It's protected to utilize this methodology on more than one occasion per week to accomplish your ideal outcomes.

Even though this procedure may appear to be simpler than curtailing day by day calories, you may get yourself very —hungry‖ on fasting days. It can likewise cause extreme symptoms or intricacies in individuals with particular wellbeing conditions.

You ought to consistently converse with your PCP before going on a fast. They can prompt you on your advantages and dangers. Continue pursuing to find out additional.

You'll be very much into your 14-hour time span before your body understands that you're fasting. During the first eight hours, your body will keep on processing your last admission of nourishment. Your body will utilize put away glucose as vitality and keep on working as if you'll be eating again soon.

After eight hours without eating, your body will start to utilize put away fats for vitality. Your body will keep on using put away fat to make vitality all through the rest of your 14-hour fast.

Fasts that last longer than 14 hours may lead to your body to begin changing over put away proteins into vitality.

24 Hour

Playing out a 24 hour fast can be a terrifying idea, yet with the correct tips and plan, you can effectively endure your fast. With this article, you will figure out how you can make it to 24 hours without breaking your fast, and find out about the advantages of fasting.

Since graduating from school, I've been hoping to try and investigate better approaches to carry on with my life without limit. Dietary patterns are one region I've concentrated on over the number of years, and specifically, trying different things with discontinuous fasting has led to some fascinating outcomes.

Regularly, I've adhered to an entirely loosened up 16-hour fasting window and 8-hour encouraging window since beginning discontinuous fasting, however now and then, I do a 24 hour fast (and once I did a 48 hour fast!)

On the off chance that you have never fasted, moving toward a 24 hour fast may appear to be a gigantic errand to take on. At the point when I began, I scarcely could make it past 9 a.m. before I –required‖ to eat. Presently, following a couple of long stretches of training, I once in a while, eat before 9 a.m.

Possibly you are interested in fasting and need to investigate your association with nourishment. It's conceivable you are hoping to get more fit and need to check whether fasting; merits giving a shot.

Whatever your explanation, I trust this post gives the data you need and need concerning fasting. Right now, I will discuss the advantages of starvation and share with your various tips for you to apply on the off chance that you are keen on a one day fast.

The Warrior Diet (The 20 Hour Fast)

The Warrior Diet is a method for eating that cycles broadened times of little nourishment admission with short windows of gorging. It has been advanced as a powerful method to get more fit and improve vitality levels and mental clearness. However, some wellbeing specialists contend that this fasting strategy is extraordinary and extravagant.

You can play out a 20-hour fast at whatever point you pick. You need to ensure that you get ready for your fasting day ahead of time. Eating healthy and balanced dinners before the fast will enable your body to traverse the 20-hour time frame.

A few nourishments you ought to consider eating preceding a fast include:

- Nourishments are wealthy in protein. For example, nut spreads and beans.
- Dairy items low in fat. For example, low-fat yogurt.
- Leafy foods.
- Entire grain starches.

Nourishments high in fiber will enable your body to feel full long in the wake of eating. Leafy foods contain water, giving you more hydration.

Drink water and other without calorie refreshments during the fast, yet remember that drinks with caffeine may make you lose more water. Drink an extra cup of water for each energized food to help balance your admission.

Keep on eating healthy after your fast is finished and abstain from indulging when it's an excellent opportunity to eat once more. You might need to have a little bite or eat a light supper when your fast finishes to assist you with moving to go into your standard eating schedule.

Alternate Day Fasting

It is a form of intermittent fasting, which involves fasting one day and eating the next and repeating this process.

A caloric limitation is a well-reported approach to get thinner, improve heart wellbeing, and conceivably even slow maturing. However, researchers, despite everything, don't concur on the ideal method to not eat.

New research in the diary Cell Metabolism plots a novel method to discontinuously confine calorie admission, a strategy that accomplishes similar medical advantages while potentially being more reasonable than continually limiting calories.

In a paper distributed on Tuesday, a worldwide group of scientists displayed the aftereffects of a clinical preliminary where –interchange day fasting‖ brought about diminished calorie admission, decreased weight record, and improved middle fat structure. Known as –ADF,‖ it is a diet routine where followers maintain a strategic distance from all nourishment and caloric drinks for 36 hours, at that point eating whatever they need for 12 hours—doughnuts, treats, dumpster pizza, whatever.

Right now, preliminary, 30 non-corpulent volunteers who had done ADF for in any event a half year were contrasted over four weeks with 60 healthy control subjects. While the consequences of this clinical preliminary show that ADF had comparative medical advantages to caloric limitation, even though the –feast days‖ could incorporate a ton of unhealthy calories. The specialists additionally compose that ADF has some unmistakable preferences over CR. For the most part, they state it might be simpler to keep up the propensity.

—Here, we appear in a clinical preliminary that a related mediation, interchange day fasting (ADF), additionally leads to a striking decrease in by and large calorie admission throughout the investigation however is more effectively endured than consistent CR and incites comparable helpful changes on the cardiovascular framework and on body piece while being ok for a time of >6 months,‖ compose the examination's creators, drove by first creator Slaven Stankovic, Ph.D., a postdoctoral scientist at the University of Graz in Austria.

—We likewise discovered positive modifications in cardiovascular illness chance variables and fat mass after just a month of ADF. Later on, this training, which is as of now developing being used as a way of life mediation, could, in the long run, oblige present-day social insurance in different settings.‖

Past work on discontinuous fasting has demonstrated that confining a creature's calories— without denying them satisfactory sustenance can expand their life expectancy. However, a significant part of the work has been constrained to monkeys and other non-human creatures.

This most recent examination expands on that current research by following a fair-sized human partner for sufficient opportunity to show critical advantages as well as no adverse symptoms.

The Two "RULES" Alternate Day Fasting

You can drink sans calorie refreshments on fasting days like unsweetened coffee and tea, water, and so forth.

You can eat up to 500 calories or 20-25% of your vitality prerequisites on fasting days.

Chapter 5

Transitioning into Intermittent Fasting (Switch Style)

Transitioning into the 16/8 Method

What Is 16/8 Intermittent Fasting?

It is not a diet; it is a type of intermittent fasting or time-restricted eating. During this, you can't only eat low calories food, but you can also eat a variety of food in this you spend 16 hours of each day consuming nothing but unsweetened beverages like water, coffee, and tea. But remaining 8, you are allowed to eat anything by doing this. You can get many benefits like you can lose your belly fat and get smarter. We should try this method every day because it's beneficial for us. Helpful fasting generally includes abandoning nourishment for a few days. On account of discontinuous fasting, then again, taking regular breaks from eating is adequate.

However, is this methodology compelling regarding the members' weight and digestion? What's more, what does science need to state about it? For numerous individuals, another year commonly implies making goals. Getting thinner is one of the most critical objectives, and there's no deficiency of chances to do as such, as counting calories methodologies flourish. Be that as it may, these frequently call for surrendering specific sorts of nourishment, a methodology that is unreasonable for some over the long haul. Interim fasting speaks to an alternate method for handling muscle versus fat. It's unique about slimming down in that it doesn't concentrate on changing what you eat, but instead basically deferring when you eat and are taking longer, regular breaks from eating.

Anna Engler found this pattern for herself and has just shed more than 30 pounds. She has been fasting utilizing the 16:8 techniques for a year now, which includes abandoning potent nourishment for 16 hours while drinking just dark espresso, tea, and water.

Eating is permitted during the remaining eight hours of the day. –I don't need to skip pizza or Turkish fringes, which are my top picks,‖ says the Berlin occupant. Engler enjoys a reprieve from eating beginning at dinnertime until lunch the next day. She says she discovers this mood to keep up, as she never especially enjoyed having breakfast in any case. For a long time, Eager struggled with low motivation, a lack of discipline, and excessive weight. The 32 years old was significantly overweight, but did not have any appetite for diets. –I always thought they were pointless because you gain back anything you have lost right away,‖ she says. ‒This seems to be a method that is relatively easy to integrate into your day to day life without causing a lot of upheavals,‖ Says Stephen Herzing. He heads up the institute for diabetes and cancer at the Zentrum vision, and he and his team conduct research into the ways that overnight fasting affects metabolism interval fasting have many other positive effects additionally to helping people reduce.

It also makes insulin more useful again, For example. Moreover, it lowers blood pressure and prevents cardiovascular disease over the long-term, and also supports cancer treatment. Together with his team, the researcher is currently exploring the questions of how fasting can be used for therapy purposes and how drugs that imitate fasting can be developed. To begin, start by picking an eight-hour window and point of confinement your nourishment admission to that time length.

Numerous individuals want to eat among early afternoon and 8 p.m., as this implies, you'll need to quick medium-term and skip breakfast yet can at present have a balanced lunch and dinner, alongside a couple of snacks for the day. Numerous people will reveal to you that it's not about the planning of your food; however, the way that you limit your food admission to an 8-hour timeframe. Yet, an ongoing examination distributed in the diary Cell Metabolism proposes that early time-limited eating (doing your fasting around evening time rather than the morning) has a medical advantage in any event when no weight reduction happens.

The examination utilized men with prediabetes and put them into two gatherings:

Early time-confined eating (6-hr nourishing period, with dinner before 3 p.m). Control bunch with a 12-hour eating plan the examination ran for five weeks. The TRF improved insulin affectability, β cell responsiveness, circulatory strain, oxidative pressure, and craving in any event when the members didn't get in shape. Be that as it may, they confined food consumption from 8 a.m. to 2 p.m. So, the examination utilized a 6-hour window rather than an 8-hour window. Remember that this methodology didn't prompt fat misfortune in all members. Fat misfortune has more to do with calorie limitation (don't accept people who reveal to you in any case) than whether you quick or not. In any case, it shows that there are medical advantages to irregular fasting/time-confined eating autonomy from weight reduction.

So, the most significant inquiry you have to answer when you follow an eating regimen or procedure like discontinuous fasting is, ‒Would I be able to make this into a way of life? On the off chance that you can't keep up an irregular fasting plan, at that point, you'll get results at first. In any case, you'll probably slide over into your old propensities as the irregular fasting plan turns out to be too difficult to even think about maintaining. The science concerning intermittent fasting is a starter and dubious because of a nonattendance of concentrates on its long-haul effects.

There is fundamental proof that discontinuous fasting might be successful for weight reduction, may diminish insulin obstruction and fasting insulin, and may improve cardiovascular and metabolic wellbeing, even though the long-haul manageability of these impacts has not been studied. The AHA suggests irregular fasting as a possibility for weight reduction and calorie control as a feature of a —purposeful way to deal with eating that centers around the planning and recurrence of dinners and snacks as the premise of a more advantageous way of life and improved hazard factor management.‖

For overweight people, fasting might be incorporated into a more extensive dietary change, for example, —putting snacks deliberately before suppers that may be related with indulging,‖ arranging dinners and snacks for the day to help oversee yearning and control feast parcels, and —advance steady medium-term quick periods.‖

The AHA noticed that eating some food on a quick day (rather than a total ready) delivered the best weight reduction and diminishes in insulin opposition when in any event, 4% weight reduction was accomplished by fat individuals. The American Diabetes Association -discovered constrained proof about the wellbeing and additionally impacts of irregular fasting on type 1 diabetes‖ and primer consequences of weight reduction for type 2 diabetes, this doesn't prescribe a particular dietary example for the administration of diabetes until more research is done, suggesting instead that —medicinal services suppliers should concentrate on the key factors that are basic among the examples.‖

New Zealand's Ministry of Health thinks about that discontinuous fasting can be advised by specialists to certain people, aside from diabetics, expressing that these —diets can be as successful as other vitality limited weight control plans, and a few people may discover them simpler to adhere to‖ yet there are conceivable symptoms during fasting days, for example, —hunger, low vitality levels, unsteadiness and poor mental working‖ and note that solid food must be picked on non-quick days.

Transitioning into 5/2

It is a type of fasting in which we eat about 25% of our total calories that are required for our bodies. Usually, we needed almost 2000 2100 calories for two days, but in this, we only consume 500 to 600 calories. When we consume low calories, it helps to reduce our weight. I am beginning the 5:2 Diet to shed a couple of pounds. We found out about it from my better half's sister, who shed more than 20 pounds in only a few months, so my significant other chose to check it out. I'm not a colossal fanatic of diets. I believe it's increasingly about –eating less and practicing more,‖ yet that doesn't appear to be working, so I wouldn't fret taking a stab at something new.

Like a decent spouse, when my significant other beginnings an eating routine, I attempt it to check whether it can work for me. Makes feast arranging a lot simpler. So, as I'm expounding on this moderately new eating regimen, I'm somewhat eager since today is one of my two low-calorie consumption days. Fundamentally, the 5:2 Diet lets you eat like you regularly accomplish for five days per week; however, then eat a low, low-calorie diet (nearly fasting) on the other two days. For my significant other, this implies only 500 calories for her and 600 calories for me. I'll get into the fundamental reasons in a minute; however, you can peruse Gina Crawford's book (and it will just take you around 30 minutes).

As indicated by Gina Crawford, Dr. Michael Mosley is the –organizer of the 5:2 Diet‖ and creator of The Fast Diet that I'm speculating broadly expounds than Ms. Crawford's guide for amateurs. Conceived in India, Dr. Mosley is currently a BBC TV columnist who produces appears on medicine and science. After a short financial vocation, Mosley chose to turn into a specialist and learned at the Royal Free Hospital Medical School. Directly after he moved on from therapeutic school in 1985, he turned into an associate maker student for the BBC. It was in 2012 that he was credited with advancing the 5:2 Diet.

The 5:2 eating routine, or The Fast Diet, is somewhat unique about most conventional, irregular fasting plans. Rather than declining food during any set fasting window, you instead drastically limit your calories for a while. In particular, you eat regularly for five days of the week. On the other two days (your decision,) ladies limit their calories to 500 for the afternoon, and men remain beneath 600 calories for each day. Genius: You never need to confront extensive periods where you're not permitted to eat anything. This is an extraordinary arrangement to slide your way into the idea of fasting, without making a plunge as far as possible. On: Two low-calorie days implies you do need to be entirely exact about checking calories two times per week, which can be a torment. That means you have to look into the caloric substance of all that you're eating, measure out your bit sizes, and keep track of the duration of the day.

Who it's for: People who appreciate the way toward tallying and following calories? (We realize you're out there!) This is additionally an extraordinary arrangement for any individual who is dismayed by the possibility of confronting cravings for food while fasting since you never really need to abandon food on this arrangement.

Monday & Thursday Fasting Days

If you choose to quickly on a Monday and a Thursday multi-week, you now need to accept to what extent you'll swoon for. You'll need ideally quick for 16 hours one after another, which has been seen as the sweet spot in fasting—you get the full advantages of a more extended fast without the challenges of finishing a more drawn out quick (contrasted with a prompt that continues for 24 hours or more).

Be that as it may, doing so might be trying with the 5:2 Diet since you separate your caloric points of confinement among breakfast and a night feast. In any case, you may think that it's more straightforward on your fasting days to get every one of your calories in a single treatment. It's truly up to you. The key is to mess with the fasting strategy for your picking; however, recollect, stick to one specific technique for a quarter of a year before you attempt another.

Wednesday & Saturday Fasting Days

By picking Wednesday and Saturday fasting days, you will not feel sincerely denied food and, subsequently, have a superior possibility of staying with the program end of the day. The 5:2 Diet is planned for getting prevent the emotions of hardship, tension, and blame that accompany such a significant number of regular diets. Fasting, no matter the technique that you pick, is never a standard eating regimen; it is a deep-rooted social change, and therefore the more you are doing it, the simpler and additionally satisfying it'll become.

The 5:2 Diet endorses two days of adjusted fasting and five days liberated from calorie tallying. When choosing which days during the week to quick, comprehend that you may be adaptable. What worked for you every week ago might not, due to social commitment or different commitments, work for you in the week?

The key is to select two nonconsecutive days during which to quick. So, as an example, on the off chance that you fasted on Monday, don't quickly again until Wednesday or later within the week, supplying you within any event one entire day between fasting periods.

Breakfast Ideas

A day of fasting may include something just like the accompanying: for breakfast, a dish (previous the toast), berries and a tablespoon of yogurt, or ¼ cup heated beans on toast. Lunch could incorporate a touch plate of mixed greens with fish, egg or grains, and dinner could be something sort of a little pan-fried food, salmon and vegetables, or another serving of mixed greens. It sounds attainable; be that because it may, nibbling within the middle of dinners would presumably set you over as far as possible, so just in case you are a slow eater, it'd be progressively troublesome.

Wolsey himself deals together with his fasting days by having a 300 Calorie breakfast at 7 a.m. (300 Calories being what could be compared to 2 cuts of light bread and a couple of bubbled eggs,) and afterward not eating again until his 300 Calorie dinner at 7 p.m.! Merely the thought of going 10 hours without eating makes my head turn, for the first part as going this era of your time without fuel makes bound to cause a make a plunge glucose levels, bringing about that trademark shakes, even as an extreme lessening in fixation and mental keenness.

Lunch Ideas

Grass-bolstered liver burgers are one among my preferred decisions for lunch during the week, and that they are incredibly simple to organize to possess during the entire week. You'll eat this over a bed of lifeless verdant greens with a primary handcrafted dressing for dinner full of B nutrients for solid methylation and detox pathways.

Dinner Ideas

Salmon may be a significant wellspring of omega-3 solid fats, and dark green veggies like kale and broccoli are high in cancer prevention agents. Salmon is one of my final top choices for its taste and supplement thickness. However, you'll choose any wild-got seafood that supported your personal preference. Serve nearby some of your preferred vegetables broiled in copra oil, and you've got a brisk and straightforward superfood feast.

Transitioning into 14/10

During a 14-hour fast, you'll expend without calorie refreshments. At the purpose when the 14-hour time-frame is finished, you'll continue your regular admission of nourishment until the subsequent fast. Notwithstanding weight misfortune, irregular fasting can positively affect your digestion, support cardiovascular wellbeing, and that is only the tip of the iceberg. It's protected to utilize this system on quite one occasion per week to accomplish your ideal outcomes.

Despite the very fact that this procedure may appear to be simpler than curtailing day by day calories, you'll get yourself very ―hungry‖ on fasting days. It can likewise cause extreme symptoms or intricacies in individuals with particular wellbeing conditions. You need to converse together with your PCP before happening quickly consistently. They will prompt you on your advantages and dangers. Continue pursuing to seek out additional. You will be considered into your 14-hour time span before your body understands that you're fasting.

During the first eight hours, your body will keep it up, processing your last admission of nourishment. Your body will utilize put away glucose as vitality and keep it up working as if you will be eating again soon. After eight hours without eating, your body will start to utilize put away fats for vitality. Your body will keep it up using put away fat to form life during the remainder of your 14-hour fast. Fasts that last longer than 14 hours may cause your body to start changing over put away proteins into energy.

Early Eating Schedule

I, for one, practice this arrangement during the weeks' worth of labor. I'm not a morning meal individual, so I appreciate a few of cups of natural tea to start my day. Despite the very fact that you merely are skipping breakfast, it's so far imperative to stay hydrated. Attempt to, in any case, drink enough water. You'll likewise have natural tea, (Most specialists concur espresso and tea don't break your quick). The catechism in tea are seemed to improve the benefits of fasting by assisting with advancing lessening the craving hormone ghrelin, so you'll cause it until lunch and to not feel denied. Since you've expanded your fasting period a further four hours, you've got to make sure your first feast (around early afternoon) has enough healthy fats. The burger within the 8-to-6-window plan will function admirably, and you'll include more fats in together with your dressing or top with avocado!

Mid-day eating schedule

Nuts and seeds make incredible tidbits that are high-fat and may be eaten around 11 a.m. Splashing these heretofore can help kill normally happening proteins like phytates, which will increase stomach related issues. Have dinner around 2:30 p.m., and quickly like within the 8-to-6-window plan, a dinner with a wild-got fish or another clean protein source with vegetables is a fantastic choice.

Evening Eating Schedule

Fat bombs will control your appetite and provides you adequate sound fats to continue you until dinner. These are particularly fulfilling in light of the very fact that they need an aftertaste like cinnamon rolls.

Transitioning into 24 Hours Fast

Playing out a 24 hour fast is often a terrifying idea, yet with the right tips and plan, you'll effectively endure your fast. With this text, you'll find out how you'll make it to 24 hours without breaking your fast, and determine the benefits of fasting. Since graduating from school, I have been hoping to undertake and investigate better approaches to hold on with my life without limit. Dietary patterns are one region I've targeting over the number of years, and specifically, trying various things with discontinuous fasting has led to some fascinating outcomes.

Regularly, I've adhered to a wholly loosened up 16-hour fasting window and eight hours encouraging window since beginning discontinuous fasting, however now then, I do a 24 hour fast (and once I did a 48 hour fast!) On the off chance that you haven't fasted, moving toward a 24 hour fast may appear to be a significant errand to require on. At the purpose, once I began, I scarcely could make it past 9 a.m. before I –required‖ to eat. Presently, following a few long stretches of coaching, I once during a while eating before 9 a.m. Possibly you're interested in fasting and wish to research your association with nourishment. It's conceivable you're hoping to urge healthier and want to see whether fasting merits giving an attempt.

Whatever your explanation, I trust this post provides the info you would like and want concerning fasting. Right now, I will be able to discuss the benefits of fasting and share with your various tips for you to use on the off chance that you are keen on a one day fast.

Additionally, called an eat-stop-eat diet, a 24-hour quick included eating no food for 24-hours one after another, typically a couple of times for each week. So you'd get fast from dinner at some point until dinner the subsequent day. Or on the opposite hand breakfast to breakfast or lunch to lunch, contingent upon what you wish. On the off chance that you erode 7 p.m. tonight and do not eat again until 7 p.m. the subsequent day, you've quite recently finished a 24-hour quick.

Professional: This one is often exceptionally like a bustling day at work. Suppose you've got a furious day at the workplace or perhaps a whole day of movement. Instead of worrying about when and what to eat amidst your confused day, enjoy a reprieve. Try not to stress overeating throughout the day, until at whatever point, you come back home for dinner.

Con: you'd prefer not to do that one consistently. It isn't prescribed to try to a 24-hour quick quite twice hebdomadally.

Who it's for: People whose bustling timetables could profit by removing the pressure of discovering, preparing, gobbling, and tidying up food for an entire day, two or three days every week. With this type of IF, you quick at some point, eat the subsequent and rehash typically. There are two or three distinct approaches to try to it – a couple of strategies permits you to eat the maximum amount as 2000 kilojoules each day on quick days, while another interchange day fasting feeds less require fast days to be no-food zones.

The weight reduction results: consistent with a recent report that contrasted exchange day fasting with standard kilojoule-limitation consumes fewer calories; the eating regimens delivered an equivalent fundamentally as weight reduction results.

Stars: Like 5:2, supporters of interchange day fasting state the break between fasting days can make this eating regimen simpler to stick to than people who require day by day kilojoule limitation.

CONS: consistent with the 2017 investigation, the inverse may be valid – more people dropped out of the opposite day fasting diet than the day kilojoule-limited one since they were disappointed with it

Since consistently day should be a fast day, paying little mind to a way of life or social duties, this sort of fasting might not be as livable as others, which can clarify the above dropout rate.

Besides, an identical report additionally found that a half year after halting the eating regimen, interchange day fasters had raised degrees of cholesterol.

What to Eat to Interrupt Your Fast?

Breaking the fast in discontinuous fasting are some things that have got to be addressed. Irregular fasting is an eating routine arrangement which incorporates fasting and eating stage in regular periods. It's viewed as compelling in accomplishing weight reduction and furnishing your body with the essential detox. Fasting stage in irregular fasting can last anyplace between 10 to 12, 14, or 16 hours, contingent upon how you are feeling. An honest fasting window keeps going anyplace between 14 to 18 hours. Way of life mentor Luke Coutinho believes that you simply ought not to drive yourself to quick longer than your body permits. Start with 10 or 12 hours at the outset and afterward expanding fasting period by an hour during a week or three days.

During the eating stage, guarantee that you devour a balanced eating routine, so you get appropriate sustenance. Likewise, it's critical to affecting bioactive food is alluded to small biomolecules that are available in foods. They need the power to balance a minimum of one metabolic procedure, which thus are often helpful for better wellbeing.

Luke's plate of incorporate bioactive papaya, pineapple, watermelon, pecans and almonds. He says that these are crude bioactive, which may give the accompanying advantages.

- Angiogenesis - a procedure which inspires arrangement of fresh recruits' vessels.
- Undifferentiated cell insurance.
- Microbiome assurance.
- DNA assurance.

As indicated by Luke, everything of the above capacities can together assist in getting a stable insusceptible system. How you break the fast in discontinuous fasting for weight reduction.

Transitioning into the Warrior Diet (The 20 Hours Fast)

The Warrior Diet may be a method for eating that cycles broadened times of little nourishment admission with short windows of gorging. It's been advanced as a reliable method to urge healthier and improve vitality levels and mental clearness. However, some wellbeing specialists contend that this fasting strategy is extraordinary and extravagant. You can play out a 20-hour fast at whatever point you choose. You merely got to make sure that you prepare for your fasting day before time. Eating healthy and balanced dinners before the fast will enable your body to traverse the 20-hour time-frame. This includes fasting for a selected measure of your time every day, at that time eating whatever you wish during the opposite 'window.'

One of the foremost documented methods for doing this is often the 16:8 eating regimen: fasting for 16 persistent hours, at that time being allowed to eat during the opposite eight, with 10 a.m.-6 p.m. the foremost generally recommended 'eating window.' The weight reduction results: An investigation distributed in 2018 found that folks following the 16:8 eating regimen lost three percent of their weight in just 12 weeks since they ate 1400 fewer kilojoules each day, on faith them. Stars: thus far, check out proposes that time-confined eating plans, for instance, 16:8 could be more straightforward to remain with than different sorts of IF, maybe in light of the very fact that you can abstain from arising to be excessively eager.

CONS: Not having the choice to eat after 6 p.m. each and each day may confine your social and family life. And keeping in mind that you could also be enticed only to postpone you're eating window once you need to, specialists caution against it for best outcomes. I would conclude that I used to be getting to awaken at 5:30 ordinarily to exercise for a fantastic remainder. It's practically smart how frequently I even have done this type of thing to tumble off the wagon following seven days. These kinds of choices and this flawlessness outlook is 100% established in dread.

On the off chance that I can control my conduct, at that time, I can control my conditions and my life. Grasping firmly to control?? Look for the dread and manage it. At the purpose, once you can remove the fear in your life, you're opened to choose positive choices toward an objective, rather than attempting to accomplish the −objective‖ in one stage. On the off chance that model? Instead of going directly from a high-sugar, throughout the day eating way of life to a 20 hour quick, perhaps venture out moving breakfast back a few hours, or dinner up a few hours.

Early Eating Schedule

Papaya and Watermelon. Papaya is the ideal natural product for weight reduction. It contains stomach related chemicals referred to as papain, which may help in facilitating pharyngitis, improving absorption, mending wounds, and decreasing muscle irritation. It's useful for people with diabetes and may likewise help in promoting menstrual pain. Watermelon comes within the classification of hydrating foods, which will forestall the lack of hydration. It's low in calories and is impeccable to be remembered for a weight reduction diet. The natural product, which is in season during summer, is plentiful in vitamin A, vitamin B6, and vitamin C. it's likewise pressed with lycopene and amino acids - which may assist you with having unbroken skin and solid invulnerability.

Mid-day eating schedule

- ½ pound ground grass-sustained meat liver.

- ½ pound ground grass-sustained meat.

- ½ teaspoon garlic powder.

- ½ teaspoon cumin powder.

- Ocean salt and pepper to taste.

- Wanted vegetable oil.

Remember that this arrangement isn't for novices, and you need to consistently converse together with your medical care physician before beginning any fasting routine, particularly on the off chance that you merely are shooting up or have an ailment. It's prescribed that espresso consumers continue their morning espresso consumption, which everybody who does propel quickly remains appropriately hydrated.

Evening Eating Schedule

Eat good fats, clean meat sources, vegetables, and a few fruits. Even however, this arrangement is propelled, it's exceptionally straightforward. Try not to eat anything one another day. Each and each other day, eat good fats, clean meat sources, vegetables, and a few organic products, and afterward, on your fasting days, you'll expend water, homegrown tea, and reasonable measures of dark espresso or tea. With this data accessible, you ought to know precisely the way to plan suppers when beginning an irregular fasting plan.

Keeping in mind that it's going to appear to be confused from the outset, once you start fasting, it'll desire natural and fit pretty flawlessly into your days. Be that because it may, consistently start slow and steadily workout to further developed plans. It's likewise imperative to remember that you may have some –off days when irregular fasting doesn't work for you. Tune to your body—on the off chance that you need to eat outside of your run of the mill window, it's OK! Restart when you are feeling much improved.

Chapter 6

Benefits, Risks and the Optimal Way of Breaking Fast

Intermittent Fasting and Its Benefits

The benefits to the brain, weight loss, and fitness make periodic fasting, an attractive option for anyone who wants to improve their health, especially for people with type 2 diabetes or those who are trying to maintain weight loss after obesity.

Slowed Aging and Improved longevity

The calorie restriction has received high pressure in the past few years for its role in increasing life expectancy in animal studies. Still, it is almost impossible to study the long-term restriction of food in humans ethically. Intermittent fasting triggers the same calorie restriction effects, so you get improved aging and a longer and healthier lifespan.

Promotes Brain Growth, Recovery, and Function

Intermittent fasting has several benefits for the brain. Tight regulation of your diet seems to improve memory, generate new neurons, improve brain recovery after an injury, raise your spirits, and reduce the risk of cognitive decline associated with aging.

Intermittent Fasting Regulates Hormone Levels

The levels of insulin, ghrelin, and leptin and the body's response improve with intermittent fasting. This means that your body is better able to respond to higher and lower blood sugar levels, as well as regulate hunger and satiety. Human growth hormone, a hormone that causes growth in children and helps regulate sugar and fat metabolism, also increases during cyclic starvation.

Intermittent Fasting Improves Blood Composition

Your body can better regulate the ebbs and flows of energy resources when you take a regular diet. Fasting, both lowering and somewhat ambiguous, helps maintain healthy blood sugar, blood pressure, insulin, and cholesterol. Improved blood composition reduces oxidative stress in the body.

Intermittent Fasting Reduces Oxidative Stress

Nutrition, as a rule, leads to oxidative stress, depletes your antioxidant defense against free radicals in your tissues. Intermittent fasting by its nature dramatically reduces your exposure to the inflammatory effects of converting food into energy because you eat less.

Intermittent Fasting Increases Fat Burning

Low insulin levels occur during fasting because you do not absorb a stable supply of glucose from the digestive tract. Low insulin levels stimulate fat-burning to maintain a steady energy level. Intermittent fasting gives you better access to your fat stores.

Intermittent Fasting Mimics the Beneficial Effects of Exercise

Sport training has many beneficial effects on the brain, heart, vascular system, stress response, and body composition. Intermittent fasting mimics many of the same benefits, such as reduced resting heart rate, improved immune function, increased DNA recovery, improved motor function, ketone production, increased stress resistance, faster recovery from stress, and enhanced disposal of old or malfunctioning cells.

Post Charts

As a rule, the longer the fasting period, the better the results. Some people find that they experience some emotional effects of fasting. You may find that you feel irritable and hot-tempered while adjusting to the intermittent fasting schedule.

Intermittent Fasting: Getting Started

If you can stretch your periodic fasting for more extended periods, you will quickly see lower levels of insulin and spend more time in ketosis, a fat-burning state.

To start intermittent fasting, we recommend starting with the 12:12 schedule: a 12-hour window where you can eat, and then a 12-hour fast. If you find this schedule simple, try program 8:16 onwards. Intermittent fasting for more extended periods with a relatively short meal period (6:18 or 4:20) is a critical component of the warrior's diet, a diet based on the eating habits of our ancestors.

Extend your post beyond this standard, and you will reach an alternative position. You must evaluate what works with your daily schedule and training goals to find a stable, steady, intermittent fasting regimen. Some fasting people think the fasting plan at 10:14 or 6:18 is better for them. In general, fasting will bring a lot of health benefits, so do not be afraid to change the schedule according to your needs. Just try to eat earlier in the afternoon and not late to reduce the accumulation of fat.

However, if you usually skip breakfast, feel free to start your meal around lunchtime. The physical impact of fasting on a person depends on innumerable variables. Some people respond to intermittent fasting significantly better than others. If you are experiencing unusual stress or experiencing some stressful life events, we would advise you to suspend your post until you cope with your weight due to the hormonal imbalance that usually accompanies (and nourishes) the reaction to stress.

Periodic Fasting - What Is During A Break?

Although you do not need to take another diet to try intermittent fasting, it is never too late to eat healthy foods. We recommend whole grains, a plant-based diet with lots of raw vegetables, fruits, nuts, and seeds to improve nutrition and maintain good health. If you want your food to contribute to fat loss, try ketogenic fasting.

Unlike most ketogenic diets or fasts, which are based on a significant amount of animal fat and protein to turn your body into ketosis, we have developed a plan to cleanse the body with whole plant foods. Such as avocados and walnuts, which contribute to healthy blood composition and reduce oxidative stress. In addition to burning fat reserves.

Does the 16/8 Diet Work?

The 16:8 diet is a type of time-restricted fasting done to achieve better health or lose weight. You will learn what the 16/8 food is and what rules you need to adhere to, losing weight in this way. The article will talk about the advantages and disadvantages of a diet, as well as how to improve the result. You will find out what you can eat on this diet and find out for how long and how many kilograms you can lose weight.

The number of diets and a variety of limiting nutritional systems is immense. Choose for every taste and color! Some are very tough and strict, such as the Japanese diet or the Maggi diet. Others are powerful and effective, such as protein or low-carb diets.

Some options are known throughout the world and by which even stars have been losing weight for many years - the Dukan diet. One way or another, there is no practical way to lose weight. No food would help everyone lose weight. Or is there any way?

Many people can involuntarily eat on the principles that will be described below. Diet 16/8 or interval diet is a way by which you do not limit yourself in any way and eat what you want, and at the same time, lose weight.

And in fact, the system is quite simple - this is the most common fasting! But the advantage is that you do not have to starve. So how does this diet work? Below you will find all the information about the principles of this method for losing weight.

Diet Rules

One way or another, before judging whether the diet will work or not, you need to understand its rules and find out why it is still so popular. The hunger strikes have long since become something completely ordinary for many people.

However, most of them do not approach this process correctly and can significantly harm their health. That is why the 16/8 diet is considered the most standard and relatively simple in the framework of the current reality. And the rules of the food are quite simple:

- Firstly, to sit on a similar diet, you must have an established schedule and sleep mode. Without this, there may not be results. Therefore, before you test your strengths through this method, think about how well you have a daily schedule. Think about what time you are most active, and what hours you rest and sleep. Based on this information, proceed to the next step.

- Next comes the most important - you choose the time for a hunger strike and the time for food. As mentioned above, you need to pick it based on your schedule. Think about what time you eat most often? Try creating a new plan so that your favorite mealtime does not disappear (even if it's the evening). But, of course, you can't eat anyway before going to bed a maximum of 2 hours before bedtime.

- An approximate graph may look as follows. You wake up at 8 o'clock, but you don't have breakfast right away. Let the body wake up, drink a glass of water on an empty stomach, take vitamins, and can-do exercises. After 2-3 hours, there will be the first meal.

- The report starts at breakfast. For example, you ate at 10 a.m., and now before 6 p.m., you will need to gain your calorie volume per day.

- After 6 pm, your fasting begins. Before going to bed, you can drink kefir or milk if you have time to get hungry, but it's better not to. With such a schedule, it is advisable to go to bed no later than 10-11 hours in the evening. Thus, you will not be hungry and will adhere to a regular sleep and diet.

Benefits

Many diets sound convincing and compelling, so most girls are always looking forward to this day with joy and embark on the active process of losing weight. But their hopes and dreams are shattered about cruel reality, because diets, especially strict ones, are crazy restrictions that neither the body nor the mind can be prepared for.

Each diet has its advantages and disadvantages. Below you will find several advantages that show this diet on the right side and can make girls think that it is beneficial and productive.

The Benefits of Diet 16/8 Are as Follows:

- Improved metabolism.
- Deep sleep.
- Stabilization of Eating Habits.
- Conscious consumption of food.
- Partially healthy nutrition.
- Lack of strict restrictions.
- Quick result.
- A simpler version for beginners (12/12, 14/10).

Disadvantages

But there are enough cons and problems with diets.

The Diet 16/8 Should Highlight the Following Disadvantages:

- Not everyone can withstand such a restrictive way to lose weight.
- Frequent hunger (first time).
- Rare but possible side effects.
- Prostration.
- Lack of mood.

- The risk of breaking and eating a lot of food in the allowed interval.

- The complexity of implementation for some people (for office workers, for example).

How to Improve Results

Of course, losing weight is a very long and complicated process, which must be approached comprehensively and wisely. Many people forget about the importance of proper nutrition on such diets, and when they see that there are —no restrictions,‖ they allow themselves to eat fast food and drink all the food. And many other things are forgotten.

- Go in for sports (moderately) and do exercises.

- To drink a lot of water.

- Do not forget that meals should be filled with proper and high-quality food.

- Do not forget about eating vegetables and fruits.

- Try to maintain good spirits and believe that you will succeed.

Dates of Diet and What Results Can Be Achieved

Above, you could already see the information that there are different options for interval fasting. Indeed, there are harder ones, for example, 18/6 hours, and more relaxed, according to which, by the way, many live without even realizing it (12 / 12, 14 / 10).

If we talk about how much you can sit on such a diet, then everyone for himself decides whether this diet will be a test period, or whether he wants to make this diet a way of his life. One way or another, you need to stop the food only if you feel bad.

How Many Calories Should You Eat On 16/8 Diet?

The rules are simple - there are any products without restrictions, but only at certain times of the day. This diet, according to American scientists, can reduce not only weight but also blood pressure. And what do our experts say?

This diet is easy to follow. Experts say this study is the first to show the benefits of full access to food at one o'clock in the day and restriction of food intake at other hours in obese people.

Researchers at the University of Illinois at Chicago studied the effects of time-limited food intake in 23 obese volunteers whose average age was 45 years old, body mass index 35 (the formula calculates body mass index (BMI) - divide centimeters by body weight in kg per squared - BMI = m / h2, the norm is up to from 18.5 to 25.5 units). The results are published in the journal Nutrition and Healthy Aging.

Participants in the study could take any food in unlimited quantities between 10.00 in the morning and 18.00. However, during the remaining 16 hours, participants could only drink water or drinks that were almost free of calories. The test lasted for 12 weeks.

Compared with the control group, participants who followed the indicated diet consumed fewer calories per day, resulting in reduced weight and blood pressure.

According to the US Centers for Disease Control and Prevention, over the past few years, more than one-third of American adults are obese. It is known that obesity significantly increases the risk of cardiovascular disease and coronary heart disease and average working age.

The average teaching art studies nick 300 kilocalories consumed less, it possible to reduce the weight to 3%, and the blood pressure at 7 mm Hg, other indicators, including body fat mass, insulin resistance, and cholesterol levels, were comparable to those in the control group.

—The main conclusion of this study is that weight loss can be made without constantly counting calories or excluding certain foods from the diet,‖ says Christa Varadi, author of the study, professor of kinesiology and nutrition.

Even though this is the first study on the 16/8 diet (16 hours of fasting and 8 hours of nutrition), Dr. Varadi notes the similarity of his results with earlier data on interval types of foods.

—The results we obtained were also observed in other studies that needed to fast for one day,‖ says Dr. Varadi, —The obvious advantage of diet 16/8 is the ease of compliance. In our study, we observed fewer dropouts due to malnutrition compared with other trials.‖

—The preliminary data obtained in the study inspire confidence, but more extensive, long-term randomized trials are required,‖ Dr. Varadi and colleagues say. —It is necessary to approach the selection of a diet individually since even a small efficiency of the method can positively affect the patient's health.‖

The opinion of The Diabetologist

The effectiveness of the 16/8 diet is related to when you go to bed.

—Such a diet will be effective only if several rules are observed,‖ says dietician Elena Solomatina. - If you go to bed late in the evening, the body will have time to get hungry and develop high levels of insulin in response to low blood glucose. And waking up in the morning, you will want to eat something sweet, flour, and high-calorie, which, due to the high level of insulin, will immediately be deposited in the tissues in the form of fat.

If you go to bed earlier, for example, at 10 p.m., you will not have time to get hungry, and in the morning, you will not be pulled for flour and sweets. In this case, this power mode will work.

But this does not mean absolute –wild freemen‖ in food. To lose weight and maintain weight at a reasonable level, it is still essential to eat the same number of calories every day, eat a balanced diet, and go to bed on time.

How Can Reduce your Stomach Fat?

A flat stomach is the ultimate dream of many women and men. The problem of fatty deposits on the abdomen is prevalent. Even with a healthy weight, you can have a tummy. It is not so simple to remove the notorious stomach, but by following our recommendations regularly, you can achieve a significant effect.

Diet to Reduce Stomach

As much as we would like, we can't do without a diet. Fat deposits in the abdomen accumulate slowly, but correctly and mainly due to an unbalanced diet. Do not be afraid of the word diet. It is not necessary to limit oneself sharply in food and refuse favorite foods; you need to revise the principles of nutrition. Fiber-rich foods contribute to volume reduction.

It absorbs excess fats and excreted from the body along with other unnecessary substances. A lot of fiber is found in fruits, vegetables, legumes, and grains. You can use thread in the form of dietary supplements. In no case, do not refuse meat. But it should not be fat, but lean (chicken, turkey, rabbit, veal).

For the meat to be well digested, it must be eaten along with vegetable salads. Do not season them with mayonnaise, it should be discarded, but olive and sunflower oil should be included in the diet. Another condition is the rejection of simple carbohydrates. It is necessary to give preference to the so-called complex carbohydrates (vegetables, fruits, rye bread, cereals, and pasta from durum wheat). But cakes, soda, chips, chocolate, and other sweets will have to be excluded—no need to abandon them altogether.

Sometimes you can afford a little of those or other –harmful‖ products. Bans more than ever negatively affect the accumulation of excess weight in our body. Another group of products that reduce volume- These are foods rich in calcium, especially dairy. Calcium helps in burning fat, and almost 80% of fat is consumed from the abdomen. And of course, liquids. Drink more water, freshly squeezed fruit and vegetable juices, decoctions of herbs.

Exercises for the Abdomen

Exercises have a good effect on reducing the volume of the abdomen. Useful exercises for the press, cardio training, aerobics, and torsion hoop. Here are a few simple, but well-proven exercises that can restore your harmony and make your stomach flat. The main rule is the regularity and correctness of their implementation.

- Exercises Cat.
- Exercises Scissors.
- Air Energy Exercises.
- Exercises Tummy Tuck.

Exercises Cat

This is a beneficial exercise; it activates many muscle groups. Sit on your palms and knees, back and arms straight, look straight ahead. Bend your back, draw in your stomach as you exhale, relax, and take a deep breath. Hold your back in an arched position for 8-10 counts. Repeat exercise 10 times.

Exercises Scissors

This exercise allows you to strengthen muscles and remove fat in the abdomen. Lie on your back, straighten your legs. Put your hands under the buttocks, palms down. The main thing to monitor the lower back, it cannot be torn off the floor. Raise your legs 10-15 cm above the level. Make broad sweeps of your legs crosswise so that one leg is above the other (scissors). Socks are elongated. The exercise is performed on 8-10 counts. Breathe smoothly, exercise methodically, and vigorously. Do not lift your feet high and pull your socks.

Air Energy Exercises

This exercise is taken from Hatha Yoga. Everyone can do this exercise; he has no contraindications. Focus on your stomach and breath. Stand straight, feet shoulder-width apart, and arms lowered along the torso. Synchronously with sharp respiration through the nose, retract the stomach as far as you can. Then, on the contrary, with a sharp breath through the nose, push the stomach as far forward as possible. This exercise for the abdomen is performed at a fast pace, carefully monitors breathing and abdominal movements, they should be simultaneous. Repeat exercise 5 times. Increase the approaches gradually, bringing their number to 25.

Exercises Tummy Tuck

Another exercise from Hatha Yoga. It is done on holding your breath. The pose is the same as in the previous training. Exhale through the nose, while pausing; tilt the upper body by 45 degrees. Hands-on hips, fingers extended to the inguinal folds, stomach drawn to the spine. Focus on the area of the solar plexus, be in such a position as you can, holding your breath.

Then relax the abdominal muscles, take a shallow, shallow breath through the nose and return to the starting position. Perform the exercise once. Once you get used to it, having trained, it can be repeated two or three times, but no more. These exercises need to be supplemented with aerobic and cardio loads. Brisk walking, jogging, training on a stationary bike, a treadmill for half an hour a day will be enough. Dancing and aerobics are great.

Massage for the Abdomen

A massage is an excellent tool in the fight against excess fat. It improves metabolism, enhances blood circulation, and improves bowel function. Together, this helps to reduce the volume of the abdomen. The main rule is that you do not need to press hard and sincerely. The main methods of massage are rubbing and kneading the skin. Grab your abdomen with your fingers and knead it intensively with your fingertips. Grab the fold either horizontally or vertically concerning the chest. Vigorous rubbing spends clockwise, using the whole hand. Twitch and shake the fat folds intensively, pinch your skin. Firmly put your palms closed in the -castle‖ to the stomach from below, raising and lowering the stomach with short sharp movements. It is better to do this while sitting or standing. Massage should be done daily for 10 minutes. To increase the effect, use anti-cellulite creams, fat-burning oils.

Water Treatment

A douche with a contrast shower will help. Contrast shower helps to increase muscle tone, increase blood circulation, and improve the overall health of the body. You can also rub the skin on the stomach and sides with a hard washcloth in circular movements until red. The changes should be significant, but soft; the pressure should be superficial.

You can massage it with a steady stream of water from the shower, directing it in a circular motion to the abdomen. A bathhouse and a steam room with a broom help well. You can take special baths with oils of orange, lemon, peppermint, sea salt while gently massaging the skin of the abdomen underwater. The procedure lasts 20 minutes. The water should be warm. After a bath, rub yourself well with a hand towel.

Chapter 7

Mindset

So, do I think it's for everybody? Honestly, and no. I unquestionably don't accept that devouring throughout the day from 6 a.m. to 10 p.m. is for anyone. A couple of people may have to start with an increasingly delicate quick, et al. could undoubtedly bounce in with none weaning period with a 23 hour a day fasting window. Takeaway? Everybody is extraordinary. There is a comic that immediately shows a specialist recommending his patient beginning gradually by fasting between dinners. That might be an honest beginning.

My mentality has changed tons, within the last 3-4 years, as I even have perused, tuned in to people's accounts, and brought responsibility to possess wellbeing. So, here are a few of the items that I also have an inclination that I should note.

Manage Stress

If you are perpetually focused on, the pressure cycle must stop. At the purpose, once I was within the downright awful sleep deprivation, and at absolutely the bottom within the excursion, I had a 1-year-old, a multi-year-old, and a multi-year old – and that they were all reception since it had been summer. Within the fall, when my most established visited Kindergarten, and my center kid and younger youngster visited preschool two days hebdomadally, I had the choice to require a couple of to urge back some composure, commit once more to figure out, and despite the very fact that I hadn't changed much else, this had a considerable effect.

Perceive the stressors throughout your life. Be straightforward on the off chance that you need a break. And do not feel terrible that or engage contemplations that you –shouldn't‖ be focused otherwise; you –should‖ have the choice to affect it. Tell the –should beast‖ to go away. You're not God, you're human, and stress is awful for you. Whatever is causing it, I make some hard memories accepting that it might ever be justified, despite all the difficulty. You'll require an opportunity, and afterward, you'll continue your way of life once you feel stable. Or not. This prompts the subsequent idea.

Be Kind to Yourself

What I mean is, approve of the way that you are not great, should not be, and you're never going to be immediate. Adding to my pressure was the way that I feel I despised myself for not having the choice to try to all the items that I figured I —SHOULD‖ have the opportunity to decide to, the smallest amount of those things being to forego dessert or a glass of wine toward the day's end. Side note: I accept wound religious philosophy added to my issues since we expect that we need to have the choice to affect hard things with God's assistance. Or on the other hand, we need to have the opportunity to prevent negative behavior patterns with God's aid.

What's more, on the off chance that we will not affect hard things or stop negative behavior patterns, we expect that this is often because we aren't asking enough or perusing enough sacred writing or serving enough, which makes us increasingly miserable and discouraged. Stop the franticness – this is not the message of the Bible. A real ramification of the gospel message is this: RELAX. The KING has come, and he LOVES you, and zip on the earth can isolate you from him. On the off chance that your —gospel‖ is prompting will-love and self-humbling, at that time, you're not confiding within the original message of the Bible. On the off chance that you can't unwind in God's unlimited love for you, at that time, you'll always be unable to satisfy his motivation for you on the world. Try not to plan to do part B without section A.

Address Your Fears

Matt always wants to ridicule me since I might —choose‖ that I might accomplish something for a mind-blowing remainder. I might conclude I used to be never getting to eat dessert again. I might find that I used to be getting to awaken at 5:30 ordinarily to exercise for a vast remainder. It's practically humorous how frequently I even have done this type of thing to tumble off the wagon following seven days. These sorts of choices and this flawless attitude are 100% established in dread. Within the event that I can control my conduct, at that time, I can control my conditions and my life.

Holding firmly to control?? Look for the dread and manage it. At the purpose, once you can eliminate the fear in your life, you're opened to choose positive choices toward an objective, rather than attempting to accomplish the -objective‖ in one stage. On the off chance that model? Instead of going directly from a high-sugar, throughout the day eating way of life to a

20-hour quick, perhaps venture out moving breakfast back a few hours, or dinner up a few hours.

One final thing: Intermittent Fasting is an instrument, yet it is not the sole device. I think it's supernatural, as you almost certainly are aware. However, everybody is extraordinary; there could be something different happening in your body that may not happen in my body—thyroid, adrenal weakness, and so on. I frequently believe that since I had likewise gotten my gut and sugar yearnings leveled out a smidgen with supplements, that it genuinely pushed my change to IF. Smart dieting is an apparatus. Enhancements are an apparatus. Fasting may be a device.

There's not a one-size-fits-all methodology, and various people are sharing what has helped them. Will it help you? I trust during this way, yet on the off chance that it doesn't, it shouldn't cause despair. I even have attempted and bombed 1000 things. This one coincidentally worked on behalf of me, and that I found it at the right time when my body and my brain were prepared for it.

Additionally, despite the very fact that I feel serene and cheerful about where I'm, I'm an extended way from great and am continually learning and evolving. Probably the foremost enlightening people I tune as to if that's podcasters, creators, or my children's teachers admit to the way that they're Always attempting to enhance. Try not to pass judgment on your excursion!